Pediatric Ultrasound Part 1

Guest Editor

BRIAN D. COLEY, MD

ULTRASOUND CLINICS

www.ultrasound.theclinics.com

October 2009 • Volume 4 • Number 4

SAUNDERS an imprint of ELSEVIER, Inc.

W.B. SAUNDERS COMPANY
A Division of Elsevier Inc.

1600 John F. Kennedy Boulevard • Suite 1800 • Philadelphia, Pennsylvania 19103-2899

http://www.theclinics.com

ULTRASOUND CLINICS Volume 4, Number 4
October 2009 ISSN 1556-858X, ISBN-13: 978-1-4160-6363-6, ISBN-10: 1-4160-6363-3

Editor: Barton Dudlick
Developmental Editor: Theresa Collier

Ultrasound Clinics (ISSN 1556-858X) is published quarterly by W.B. Saunders, 360 Park Avenue South, New York, NY 10010-1710. Months of publication are January, April, July, and October. Business and editorial offices: 1600 John F. Kennedy Boulevard, Suite 1800, Philadelphia, Pennsylvania 19103-2899. Accounting and circulation offices: 6277 Sea Harbor Drive, Orlando, FL 32887-4800. Periodicals postage paid at New York, NY, and additional mailing offices. Subscription prices are $189 per year for (US individuals), $274 per year for (US institutions), $94 per year for (US students and residents), $215 per year for (Canadian individuals), $306 per year for (Canadian institutions), $229 per year for (international individuals), $306 per year for (international institutions), and $114 per year for (Canadian and foreign students/residents). To receive student/resident rate, orders must be accompanied by name of affiliated institution, date of term, and the signature of program/residency coordinator on institution letterhead. Orders will be billed at individual rate until proof of status is received. Foreign air speed delivery is included in all Clinics subscription prices. All prices are subject to change without notice. **POSTMASTER:** Send address changes to *Ultrasound Clinics,* Elsevier Health Sciences Division, Subscription Customer Service, 3251 Riverport Lane, Maryland Heights, MO 63043. **Customer Service (orders, claims, online, change of address): Telephone: 1-800-654-2452 (U.S. and Canada); 314-447-8871(outside U.S. and Canada). Fax: 314-447-8029. E-mail: journalscustomerservice-usa@elsevier.com (for print support); journalsonlinesupport-usa@elsevier.com (for online support).**

Reprints: For copies of 100 or more, of articles in this publication, please contact the Commercial Reprints Department, Elsevier Inc., 360 Park Avenue South, New York, NY 10010-1710. Tel.: (+1) 212-633-3812; Fax: (+1) 212-462-1935; E-mail: reprints@elsevier.com.

Contributors

GUEST EDITOR

BRIAN D. COLEY, MD
Department of Radiology, Nationwide
Children's Hospital, Columbus, Ohio; Clinical
Professor of Radiology and Pediatrics, The
Ohio State University College of Medicine
and Public Health, Columbus, Ohio

AUTHORS

LYNN ANSLEY FORDHAM, MD
Associate Professor, Department of Radiology,
School of Medicine, University of North Carolina,
Chapel Hill, North Carolina; Chief, Division of
Pediatric Imaging, North Carolina Children's
Hospital, UNC Hospitals, North Carolina

LORI L. BARR, MD
Adjunct Associate Professor of Radiology,
Department of Radiology, The University of
Texas Medical Branch, Galveston; Partner,
Austin Radiology Association, Austin, Texas

DOROTHY I. BULAS, MD
Professor of Pediatrics and Radiology,
Department of Diagnostic Imaging and
Radiology, Children's National Medical Center,
George Washington University Medical Center,
Washington, DC

MICHAEL A. DIPIETRO, MD
John F. Holt Collegiate Professor of Radiology,
Department of Radiology, C.S. Mott Children's
Hospital, University of Michigan, Ann Arbor,
Michigan

JOSÉE DUBOIS, MSc, MD, FRCP(C)
Clinical Professor of Radiology, Department
of Radiology, Radio-Oncology and Nuclear
Medicine, University of Montreal; Chief,
Department of Medical Imaging, CHU
Sainte-Justine Mother and Child University
Hospital Center, Montreal, Quebec, Canada

NANCY R. FEFFERMAN, MD
Assistant Professor of Radiology, Section
Chief, Division of Pediatric Radiology,
Department of Radiology, New York
University Langone Medical Center,
New York, New York

MARIA F. LADINO TORRES, MD
Clinical Lecturer, Department of Radiology,
C.S. Mott Children's Hospital, University
of Michigan, Ann Arbor, Michigan

LISA H. LOWE, MD
Professor Pediatric Radiology, Department
of Radiology, University of Missouri-Kansas
City School of Medicine, Children's Mercy
Hospitals and Clinics, Kansas City,
Missouri

OSCAR M. NAVARRO, MD
Associate Professor, Department of Medical
Imaging, University of Toronto; Department
of Diagnostic Imaging, The Hospital for Sick
Children, Toronto, Ontario, Canada

KAY NORTH, DO
Fellow Pediatric Radiology, Department
of Radiology, University of Missouri-Kansas
City School of Medicine, Children's Mercy
Hospitals and Clinics, Kansas City,
Missouri

DIMITRI A. PARRA, MD
Assistant Professor, Department of Medical
Imaging, University of Toronto; Division
of Image Guided Therapy, Department
of Diagnostic Imaging, The Hospital
for Sick Children, Toronto, Ontario,
Canada

FRANÇOISE RYPENS, MD
Clinical Associate Professor of Radiology,
Department of Radiology, Radio-Oncology

and Nuclear Medicine, University of Montreal;
Staff Radiologist, Department of Medical
Imaging, CHU Sainte-Justine Mother and
Child University Hospital Center, Montreal,
Quebec, Canada

SARAH SARVIS MILLA, MD
Assistant Professor of Radiology, Division
of Pediatric Radiology, Department of
Radiology, New York University Langone
Medical Center, New York, New York

Contents

This article describes the use of ultrasound for detecting abnormalities in the heads of infants. The authors provide guidance on how to distinguish normal structures, variants, and image artifacts from true abnormalities. While ultrasound has its limitations, recent studies comparing magnetic resonance imaging and computed tomography to careful head sonogram have shown that, for detecting abnormalities, ultrasound offers the accuracy required to make an initial diagnosis and guide management. Ultrasound has the benefit of being portable, which means it may be performed at the bedside of unstable infants who cannot safely be brought to radiology for other neuroimaging. In addition, ultrasound does not expose the infant to radiation and is less expensive than other imaging modalities.

Neurosonography remains the preferred method of early imaging of the brain while the fontanelles remain open because of low cost, portability, and safety. This article provides a framework for expansion of one's ability to detect the gamut of neuropathology affecting infants through various applications of neurosonography. In all conditions—congenital, infectious, neoplastic, and injury—neurosonography is often the first step. With 3-dimensional localization, advances in quantitative algorithms, and forays into ultrasound contrast administration, additional value may be obtained in the future from this bedside modality.

Transcranial Doppler can be a useful tool in the assessment of intracranial abnormalities both in the neonate and child. Transcranial Doppler has become important in the management of children with sickle cell anemia. It can be used to assess asphyxia, hydrocephalus, vascular malformations, vasospasm, and brain death in infant, children and adults. This article describes the technique, safety, Doppler measurements, and abnormal cerebral hemodynamics of transcranial Doppler applications in neonates and children.

Lesions involving the pediatric neck are common and may involve any of the soft tissue, vascular, or osseous structures contained within this space. Imaging evaluation of the neck in children can be challenging. Computed tomography and magnetic resonance imaging provide excellent spatial resolution and superior tissue contrast, respectively, but have inherent limitations if used in children. Ultrasound provides a relatively risk-free, rapid, noninvasive imaging modality that is particularly useful in children. Ultrasound has been accepted as an effective means of imaging the neck in children for a variety of indications, including the initial evaluation of palpable masses and conditions affecting the thyroid gland. This article examines the use of ultrasound in the imaging evaluation of pediatric neck abnormalities.

Ultrasound Clinics

THE CLINICS ARE NOW AVAILABLE ONLINE!

Access your subscription at:
www.theclinics.com

GOAL STATEMENT

The goal of the *Ultrasound Clinics* is to keep practicing radiologists and radiology residents up to date with current clinical practice in ultrasound by providing timely articles reviewing the state of the art in patient care.

ACCREDITATION

The *Ultrasound Clinics* is planned and implemented in accordance with the Essential Areas and Policies of the Accreditation Council for Continuing Medical Education (ACCME) through the joint sponsorship of the University of Virginia School of Medicine and Elsevier. The University of Virginia School of Medicine is accredited by the ACCME to provide continuing medical education for physicians.

The University of Virginia School of Medicine designates this educational activity for a maximum of 15 *AMA PRA Category 1 Credits*™ for each issue, 60 credits per year. Physicians should only claim credit commensurate with the extent of their participation in the activity.

The American Medical Association has determined that physicians not licensed in the US who participate in this CME activity are eligible for a maximum of 15 *AMA PRA Category 1 Credits*™ for each issue, 60 credits per year.

Credit can be earned by reading the text material, taking the CME examination online at http://www.theclinics.com/home/cme, and completing the evaluation. After taking the test, you will be required to review any and all incorrect answers. Following completion of the test and evaluation, your credit will be awarded and you may print your certificate.

FACULTY DISCLOSURE/CONFLICT OF INTEREST

The University of Virginia School of Medicine, as an ACCME accredited provider, endorses and strives to comply with the Accreditation Council for Continuing Medical Education (ACCME) Standards of Commercial Support, Commonwealth of Virginia statutes, University of Virginia policies and procedures, and associated federal and private regulations and guidelines on the need for disclosure and monitoring of proprietary and financial interests that may affect the scientific integrity and balance of content delivered in continuing medical education activities under our auspices.

The University of Virginia School of Medicine requires that all CME activities accredited through this institution be developed independently and be scientifically rigorous, balanced and objective in the presentation/discussion of its content, theories and practices.

All authors/editors participating in an accredited CME activity are expected to disclose to the readers relevant financial relationships with commercial entities occurring within the past 12 months (such as grants or research support, employee, consultant, stock holder, member of speakers bureau, etc.). The University of Virginia School of Medicine will employ appropriate mechanisms to resolve potential conflicts of interest to maintain the standards of fair and balanced education to the reader. Questions about specific strategies can be directed to the Office of Continuing Medical Education, University of Virginia School of Medicine, Charlottesville, Virginia.

The faculty and staff of the University of Virginia Office of Continuing Medical Education have no financial affiliations to disclose.

The authors/editors listed below have identified no professional or financial affiliations for themselves or their spouse/partner:
Lori L. Barr, MD; Matthew J. Bassignani, MD (Test Author); Dorothy I. Bulas, MD; Brian D. Coley, MD (Guest Editor); Michael A. DiPietro, MD; Josée Dubois, MSc, MD, FRCP(C); Barton Dudlick (Acquisitions Editor); Nancy R. Fefferman, MD; Lynn Ansley Fordham, MD; Lisa H. Lowe, MD; Sarah Sarvis Milla, MD; Oscar M. Navarro, MD; Kay North, DO; Dimitri A. Parra, MD; Françoise Rypens, MD; and Maria F. Ladino Torres, MD.

Disclosure of Discussion of Non-FDA Approved Uses for Pharmaceutical Products and/or Medical Devices.
The University of Virginia School of Medicine, as an ACCME provider, requires that all faculty presenters identify and disclose any off-label uses for pharmaceutical and medical device products. The University of Virginia School of Medicine recommends that each physician fully review all the available data on new products or procedures prior to clinical use.

TO ENROLL

To enroll in the Ultrasound Clinics Continuing Medical Education program, call customer service at 1-800-654-2452 or visit us online at www.theclinics.com/home/cme. The CME program is available to subscribers for an additional fee of $205.00.

Preface

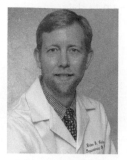

Brian D. Coley, MD
Guest Editor

Since the last pediatric issue of *Ultrasound Clinics*, a lot of attention has been paid to medical radiation exposure, especially in children. Ultrasound has always been valuable for imaging children, but even in pediatric radiology there has been a gradual drift toward computed tomography for many clinical situations. Fortunately, attitudes may be changing again with ultrasound coming back into favor. Computed tomography is a terrific modality and absolutely vital to modern medical practice. However, many cases are as well evaluated with ultrasound, which may often be the preferable modality. Ultrasound is the ultimate way to "image gently." Our nonradiology colleagues have increasingly recognized the value of ultrasound, and its use has risen dramatically among these clinicians (generally to the concern and consternation of radiologists). Some of this is inevitable as equipment becomes better, smaller, and cheaper. Some of this, unfortunately, is due to the abandonment of ultrasound by radiologists and the diminished ultrasound educational experience provided by many of our training programs.

To really appreciate the value of ultrasound, you have to hold a transducer, put some gel on a patient, and do some scanning yourself. The articles in this issue are all written by excellent sonologists with practical experience in using ultrasound as a clinical problem-solving tool in pediatrics. Because many people are nervous

approaching a sick child, we start the issue with useful advice about how to put the patient and family (and the sonographer) at ease to successfully complete an examination. The remainder of this issue focuses on musculoskeletal applications; on applications related to the brain, head, and neck; and on applications concerning vascular malformations. A subsequent issue will cover abdominal and pelvic topics. Barton Dudlick and the staff at Elsevier remain a pleasure to work with, and I appreciate the care that they have taken in the preparation of the material. I offer my thanks to the authors on the terrific material they have assembled, and I know how hard it can be to find time in a busy practice to write. We will all be better pediatric imagers for their efforts.

Brian D. Coley, MD
Department of Radiology
Nationwide Children's Hospital
700 Children's Drive
Columbus, OH 43205, USA

The Ohio State University College of
Medicine and Public Health
Columbus, OH, USA

E-mail address:
Brian.Coley@nationwidechildrens.org

Ultrasound Clin 4 (2009) ix
doi:10.1016/j.cult.2009.11.008

Approach to the Pediatric Patient

Lynn Ansley Fordham, MD[a,b,*]

KEYWORDS

- Pediatric sonography • Pediatric ultrasound exam
- Developmental approach • Age appropriate
- Infant • Toddler • Child

Working with children can be very challenging. Pediatric patients are challenging because of the wide range in ages and developmental abilities. The approach one takes to the premature infant is very different from the approach to the surly teenager. Working with children can be very rewarding, as a positive interaction and a correct diagnosis can have repercussions for the child and the child's family for years to come. Unfortunately, negative interactions can also be remembered for years. The memory of a negative encounter can make the next visit to the ultrasound department that much more difficult for the child, the family, and the sonologist. An understanding of some of the central theories of child development, coupled with awareness of the more general issues in working with children can lead to a win-win-win situation. Namely, an efficiently acquired high-quality examination obtained in a low-stress, pleasant environment in which the patient, the parents, and the sonographer can all be proud of the study and how it was accomplished. In this article we review an age-stratified approach to working with children and their families. Socioeconomic factors and cultural backgrounds also factor into the sonographer-patient-family interaction, but these are outside the scope of this article, although many excellent resources are available in this area.[1–4]

THEORETICAL MODELS OF CHILD DEVELOPMENT

There are many different ways to look at child development. Freud, Erikson, and Piaget are all famous names in the realm of child psychology and human development. They have differing theories, but all look at development as a process through which all healthy normal children progress. An understanding of these theoretical frameworks can lead to insight into the meaning of behaviors observed in individual children and to their reactions and perceptions of their experience in the ultrasound department. Each of these researchers has published extensively and so only a brief synopsis can be presented here. A hybrid combination of these theories seems to be most useful in the clinical realm.[1]

One of the first theories to be proposed was the maturational theory-normative approach. In this theoretical framework, the child progresses sequentially through developmental milestones. In this model psychological development is linked to physical development. A child's psychological development can then be compared against age-based norms.[1]

Freud took a different approach.[1,4] He described the importance of early childhood experience in adult life. He believed unconscious processes were important in shaping behavior as is the relationship between caregiver and child. Freud divides the self into three categories: the id, the ego, and the superego. In the Freudian model, the child works through a series of psychosexual conflicts. The conflicts are between inner desires and the external world. Successful resolutions of the conflicts lead ultimately to successful separation from the parent/caregiver. Freud

a Department of Radiology, School of Medicine, University of North Carolina, Campus Box #7510, Chapel Hill, NC 27599-7510, USA
b Division of Pediatric Imaging, North Carolina Children's Hospital, UNC Hospitals, NC, USA
* Department of Radiology, School of Medicine, University of North Carolina, Campus Box #7510, Chapel Hill, NC 27599-7510.
E-mail address: fdh@med.unc.edu

Ultrasound Clin 4 (2009) 439–443
doi:10.1016/j.cult.2009.10.002

describes the following five stages of development:

1. Oral phase (infancy to 18 months) where the central theme is feeding
2. Anal phase (18 months to 3 years) focusing on elimination
3. Phallic stage (3–6 years) identification of sexual self
4. Latency period (6–11 years) increasing control over sexual drive and aggression
5. Genital stage (12 years–adult) development of relationships outside family.

Erik Erikson also divided childhood into five stages, each with a conflict to be resolved. The central conflicts in his psychosocial theory are outlined as follows[1,5]:

1. Trust versus mistrust (infancy to 18 months)
2. Autonomy versus shame and doubt (18 months to 3 years)
3. Initiative versus guilt (3–6 years)
4. Industry versus inferiority (6–11 years)
5. Identity versus role confusion (adolescence).

In both the Freudian psychosexual theory and the Erikson psychosocial theory, the inner emotional life of the child is the major factor in the development of the child.

Behaviorism and social learning theory[1] both view the environment as the major force shaping a child. In behaviorism, the behavior of a child is rewarded or punished by the environment and therefore certain behaviors are encouraged whereas others are discouraged. Social learning theory builds on behaviorism with the addition of modeling of good behaviors and in role playing to practice positive behaviors.

In the constructivist theory of Piaget,[1] cognitive development depends on both the child and the surrounding environment. The child experiments, interacts with, and learns from the environment and uses the new knowledge to refine his or her behaviors to then interact in more complex ways. The following are the four stages of development in this system:

1. Sensorimotor (birth to 2 years): understands the world through direct sensation and actions
2. Preoperational (2 to 6 years): understands the world through own perceptions with no separation between internal and external reality
3. Concrete operational (6–11 years): uses reason to understand rules
4. Formal operational (12–adult): able to think abstractly considering ideas, possibilities, and probabilities.

In addition to developmental stages, patient temperament also has an important impact on the patient experience. Temperament is defined as those stable, individual differences in emotional reactivity, activity level, attention, and self-regulation.[1] There are nine dimensions of temperament. These can be assessed formally but for our purpose are assessed informally. These factors are activity level, rhythmicity, response to new stimuli (approach vs withdrawal), adaptability, attention span, distractibility, intensity of reaction, threshold of responsiveness, and overall mood. A quick assessment of patient and family temperament can help sonographers match their style of interaction and help make the patient and family comfortable and vice versa. A well-meaning but boisterous sonographer can frighten a shy child and make it difficult to obtain a full examination.

PRACTICAL APPLICATIONS

Understanding the fundamental points in these differing theories of child development and combining this with the physiologic developmental milestone can help to tailor the approach to different age children. This is summarized in **Table 1**.[1,6] For example, a 3-year-old may be motivated to cooperate for an ultrasound examination by a combination of praise for being a "big girl" and pretend play with the "magic wand" of the ultrasound transducer. The school-age child may respond well to a concrete explanation and to being given a job such as holding "really still" as part of the ultrasound examination. Concrete rewards such as stickers and verbal rewards in the form of praise help to make the experience an enjoyable one. Conversely, a 4-year-old left alone in the darkened examination room for even a moment may interpret the experience as abandonment and punishment for being bad.[6–9]

There are a few features that are important for all children visiting the ultrasound department. The check-in process should be easy and friendly. The waiting room should be bright and comfortable. The staff should be friendly and efficient, and the focus should always be on the child. If the staff does not speak the family's language, an interpreter should be contacted quickly. Whenever possible, children should wait in a separate waiting area decorated in a child-friendly manner stocked with age-appropriate distractions such as washable toys, coloring pages and take-home crayons, a variety of books and magazines, and a television set to a channel appropriate for all in the waiting room.[4,7] Video games can also be a bonus but few children like to be interrupted in

Table 1
Age-based approach to the ultrasound examination

Age (Approximate)	Developmental Stage	Approach to Sonographic Examination
Birth to 6 months (Infant)	Symbiotic (does not fear strangers)	Examine infant on examination table or parent's lap doing easiest parts of examination first
6 months to 3 years (Toddler)	Separation-individuation (fear of strangers, toddler clings to parent)	Perform examination while parent holding (in lap, lying on chest, etc); peekaboo games and toys to distract
3–6 years (Preschooler)	Age of initiation (fantasy play, increasing verbal ability)	Talk to child and explain procedure in simple language, ask the child to participate, take advantage of child's ability to pretend both for distraction and cooperation
6–12 years (School age)	Age of industry (increasing knowledge, increased understanding of cause and effect)	Explain the reasons for the procedure, the procedure, and the results in simple language; understanding improves cooperation
12–19 years (Adolescent)	Age of identity (increased awarness of self and effect on others)	Increased ability to understand procedures and implications Increased autonomy Respect for patient privacy vital

Data from Colarusso CA. Psychological approach to the pediatric patient. In: Edwards DK III, Hilton SVW, editors. Practical pediatric radiology. 3rd edition. Philadelphia: Saunders Elsevier; 2006. p. 642; Dixon SD, Stein MT. Encounters with children: pediatric behavior and development. St Louis (MO): Mosby; 2000.

the middle of a game. The child should be examined in a room with a friendly, cheerful décor. There should be a balance struck so that the furnishings aren't too babyish but still appeal to the younger children. A television with a DVD player and a selection of movies and prerecorded shows also helps to pass the time amiably. Children who visit frequently can be invited to bring their own DVDs or toys. The temperature in the rooms should be warm enough so that the partially disrobed child is comfortable. This is higher for babies than older children. Unless there is a special request for a tour, children should be shielded from the work areas of the department where they might misinterpret what they observe or simply feel ignored. There are many sources of information that offer suggestions on working with children.[1,5–13] The following sections can serve as an outline for age-specific modifications to the ultrasound examination.

1. Infancy
   a. Allow parent to remain with the infant throughout the procedure to avoid feelings of abandonment. If a parent is not available, a surrogate should be appointed.
   b. A pacifier, gentle repetitive noises or motions, and singing or soft music can all help to sooth an infant.
   c. Avoid sudden loud noises or changes in lighting that may startle the infant.
2. Toddler
   a. Allow parent to remain with the child.
   b. Allow child to explore the examination room and be active.
   c. Distraction games such as peekaboo can be helpful.
3. Preschool
   a. Allow the parent to remain with the child and participate.
   b. Explain the examination in simple language and answer all questions honestly.
   c. Magic and pretend can be used to make the examination more fun and to elicit cooperation. If a child can't hold his or her breath on command, he or she may be able to pretend to blow bubbles and accomplish the same goal.

d. Respect the child's modesty by pulling curtains, shutting doors, and by only uncovering areas to be examined.

4. School age
   a. Parental presence is optional and will depend on the type of examination and the individual child.
   b. This age group generally admires, respects, and trusts adults. They expect to be taken seriously and have the procedure and "rules" fully explained in great detail. They resent any omission or deviation from what was explained.
   c. The child can be enlisted as an ally or given a task to perform to facilitate the examination.
   d. Give them choices and let them make some decisions to maintain control.
   e. Respect for modesty becomes more important.

5. Adolescence
   a. Respect for patient modesty and privacy essential.
   b. Parents are not present in the examination room unless requested by the child. A chaperone and same sex sonographer may be helpful depending on the type of the examination.
   c. Treat adolescents with same level of dignity and respect as you would an adult both in explaining the examination and the results.

THE SICK CHILD

A child's response to illness, like the response to the ultrasound examination, will depend on his or her developmental level. Similar to adults, sick children may become withdrawn with decreased levels of activity and decreased interest in people, play, or their surroundings.[1,6] Children can also become aggressive and act out or regress back to an earlier developmental stage.[4,7] Children with chronic illness have likely had a prior ultrasound examination and their reaction with be modulated by the earlier experience. Likewise, children may be anticipating a painful procedure or they may be anxious about the results of their test. Remember, the family of the sick child is also experiencing stress. They may be anxious, depressed, sleep deprived, or distracted because of financial concerns or worries about the patient or other family members. They may not listen to or understand the explanations given. A calm, warm, caring environment and patient-focused examination will not only help the child, but will also help to minimize the stress experienced by the caregiver.

THE CHILD WITH DISABILITIES

Children can be disabled because of acute or chronic conditions. Disabilities can be primarily cognitive or physical. A child can have a single or multiple disabilities. A team approach to these children and their families can be very helpful.[3] Allow extra time for the examination. Taking a few moments to review prior ultrasound examinations and to review the medical record can help streamline the current examination and help the sonographer know what to expect and which areas to focus on so that the most important images are obtained first.

THE DYING CHILD

This topic is a difficult one for all who are involved in the care of children.[3,4,7,14] A child-centered approach is required with recognition of and sensitivity to the added stress experienced by the child and the family. As a care provider and member of the team, it is also important to recognize and acknowledge one's own feelings so that they don't interfere with patient care.

SUMMARY

Children are unique individuals who share certain commonalities based on age, temperament, and developmental stage. Planning and age-appropriate interactions can make the ultrasound examination a positive experience for all involved.

REFERENCES

1. Dixon SD, Stein MT. Encounters with children: pediatric behavior and development. St. Louis (MO): Mosby; 2000.
2. Walker S. Culturally competent therapy: working with children and young people. New York: Palgrave Macmillan; 2005.
3. Beckman PJ. Strategies for working with families of young children with disabilities. Baltimore: P.H. Brookes Pub. Co; 1996.
4. Levine MD, Carey WB, Crocker AC. Developmental-behavioral pediatrics. 3rd edition. Philadelphia: Saunders; 1999.
5. Carey WB. Developmental-behavioral pediatrics. 4th edition. Philadelphia: Saunders/Elsevier; 2009.
6. Colarusso CA. Psychological approach to the pediatric patient. In: Edwards DK III, Hilton SVW, editors. Practical pediatric radiology. 3rd edition. Philadelphia: Saunders Elsevier; 2006. p. 642.
7. Center for Attitudinal Healing. Advice to doctors & other big people from kids. Berkeley (CA): Celestial Arts; 1991.

8. Powers SW. Empirically supported treatments in pediatric psychology: procedure-related pain. J Pediatr Psychol 1999;24:131.

9. Stephens BK, Barkey ME, Hall HR. Techniques to comfort children during stressful procedures. Accid Emerg Nurs 1999;7:226.

10. Cohen LL, Blount RL, Panopoulos G. Nurse coaching and cartoon distraction: an effective and practical intervention to reduce child, parent, and nurse distress during immunizations. J Pediatr Psychol 1997;22:355.

11. Dowling JS. Humor: a coping strategy for pediatric patients. Pediatr Nurs 2002;28:123.

12. Peterson L. Coping by children undergoing stressful medical procedures: some conceptual, methodological, and therapeutic issues. J Consult Clin Psychol 1989;57:380.

13. Volkl-Kernstock S, Felber M, Schabmann A, et al. Comparing stress levels in children aged 2–8 years and in their accompanying parents during first-time versus repeated voiding cystourethrograms. Wien Klin Wochenschr 2008; 120:414.

14. Hill L. Caring for dying children and their families. London: Chapman & Hall; 1994.

Developmental Dysplasia of the Hip

Maria F. Ladino Torres, MD[a,*], Michael A. DiPietro, MD[b]

KEYWORDS

- Developmental dysplasia of the hip
- Ultrasound • Congenital

Ultrasound is widely used to assess the infant hip in the evaluation of developmental dysplasia of the hip (DDH), formerly referred to as congenital dislocation of the hip. DDH includes the spectrum of this condition with its range of abnormality and changes over time. Ultrasound evaluation of the cartilaginous and osseous components of the young infant hip at rest and during dynamic maneuvers provides information about morphology, position, and stability.

BACKGROUND

Developmental dysplasia of the hip includes a spectrum of abnormalities ranging from slightly subluxated to markedly dislocated hips. The dysplastic hip could manifest mild joint laxity or irreducible dislocation. In utero, normal hip development involves a close association and congruency between the growing femoral head and the acetabulum. Acetabular dysplasia could be the initial abnormality or it could be secondary to in utero hip subluxation. Physiologic, mechanical, and genetic factors are implicated in DDH. Physiologically, maternal hormones near delivery produce a temporary laxity of the hip joint. Mechanically, constant compression in utero with spatial restriction of movements is accentuated in late gestation, with first pregnancy, oligohydramnios, and breech presentation. Other conditions associated with in utero constraint, such as sternocleidomastoid torticollis (fibromatosis colli); foot deformities (ie, metatarsus adductus, clubfoot); and molding deformity of the skull, have an increased

association with DDH. Genetically, DDH is more likely with a positive family history and among certain ethnic populations.[1–3]

Newborn physiologic hip-joint laxity with or without a slightly immature acetabulum that resolves spontaneously by 6 to 8 weeks is considered the mildest end of the DDH spectrum. Based on the position of the femoral head and its stability within the acetabulum, the hip is described as subluxatable, subluxated relocatable, subluxated irreducible, dislocatable, dislocated reducible, or as dislocated irreducible. Acetabular dysplasia can exist with or without joint laxity and is also a part of DDH. DDH is a treatable condition and is treated successfully when intervention begins early. Therefore early detection is essential.

In DDH, the hip is rarely frankly dislocated at birth. Teratologic hip dysplasia is a special category of dislocation seen in newborn babies with an underlying neuromuscular condition, such as myelomeningocele or caudal regression syndrome, in which the hip is dislocated early in gestation leading to advanced acetabular and femoral changes, such as a pseudoacetabulum being present at birth.[3]

The incidence of DDH before clinical screening programs was reported to be between 0.07% and 0.15% of live births, whereas after clinical screening programs it was reported to be between 0.25% and 2% of live births. However, the rate of late diagnosed cases was no different; the apparent increase in the incidence of DDH with clinical screening could merely be a difference in classification, including many patients who might have recovered spontaneously without treatment.[4]

[a] Department of Radiology, C.S. Mott Children's Hospital, University of Michigan, Room F3345, 1500 East Medical Center Drive, Ann Arbor, MI 48109-5252, USA
[b] Department of Radiology, C.S. Mott Children's Hospital, University of Michigan, Room 3351, 1500 East Medical Center Drive, Ann Arbor, MI 48109-5252, USA
* Corresponding author.
E-mail address: marialad@med.umich.edu (M.F. Ladino Torres).

Ultrasound Clin 4 (2009) 445–455
doi:10.1016/j.cult.2009.11.004
1556-858X/09/$ – see front matter © 2009 Elsevier Inc. All rights reserved.

ULTRASOUND

Ultrasound displays the cartilaginous components of the femoral head, the acetabulum, the labrum, and the joint capsule. The newborn femoral head and greater trochanter are entirely cartilaginous. The acetabulum has cartilaginous and ossified components. The osseous acetabulum is formed by portions of the ilium, ischium, and pubis, which join at their growth cartilage, the triradiate cartilage. The acetabulum, femoral head, and greater trochanter hyaline cartilage appear hypoechoic with multiple low-level echoes caused by vascular channels. This hyaline cartilage will eventually ossify. In contrast, the joint capsule is echogenic and attaches to the femoral metaphysis and to the acetabulum peripheral to the labrum. The osseous femoral metaphysis and ossified components of the acetabulum produce brightly reflecting echoes. Although the entire unossified acetabular roof is sometimes referred to as the labrum, the echogenic fibrocartilage of the edge of the cartilaginous roof is the true labrum.

The ossification center of the femoral head appears radiographically between the sixth week and the eighth month of postnatal life and is seen earlier in girls than in boys. The ossification center in the developing femoral head is visible sonographically as a central echogenicity before it appears radiographically. Later in infancy the size of the ossification center hinders sonographic visualization of the acetabulum.[5]

Using ultrasound one can reliably assess hip-joint morphology and stability. Ultrasound techniques of Graf and Harcke are most often used in combination. The initial work of Graf[6] focused on acetabular morphology of the hip joint from a standard coronal plane through the mid acetabulum.[7] The hip is classified as one of four main types (from physiologic immaturity to marked dysplasia) based on the osseous acetabular modeling, the cartilaginous acetabular rim, the osseous acetabular roof inclination angle (α angle), and the cartilaginous acetabular roof angle (β angle). Harcke began using a dynamic real-time scanning approach based on coronal and transverse views of the hip in neutral and flexed positions, including a description of hip stability during stress similar to the physical examination.[8,9] Although many radiologists had already combined the two methods, Drs. Harcke and Graf[10] proposed a standard minimum examination of the hip including examining at rest in the coronal plane and in transverse plane during stress maneuvers.[11]

The American College of Radiology (ACR) published a standard for assessment of the infant hip. The examination requires evaluation of the

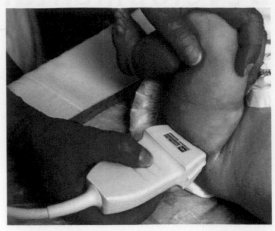

Fig. 1. Picture illustrating the position of the hip and transducer to obtain a coronal view. (*From* DiPietro MA, Harcke T. Pediatric musculoskeletal and spinal sonography. In: van Holsbeeck MT, Introcaso JH, editors. Musculoskeletal ultrasound. 3rd edition. Philadelphia: Mosby; 2010.)

relationship of the femoral head to the acetabulum on two orthogonal planes, coronal view in standard plane at rest, and transverse view of the flexed hip at rest and during stress maneuvers (position and stability). Morphology is assessed at rest, and the stress maneuvers follow the clinic examination maneuvers to assess for femoral stability.[12–14]

TECHNIQUE

A real-time linear array transducer is recommended with the highest frequency that allows

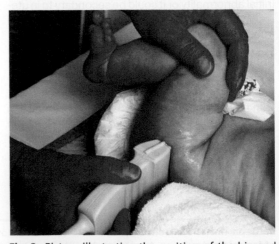

Fig. 2. Picture illustrating the position of the hip and transducer to obtain a transverse view. (*From* DiPietro MA, Harcke T. Pediatric musculoskeletal and spinal sonography. In: van Holsbeeck MT, Introcaso JH, editors. Musculoskeletal ultrasound. 3rd edition. Philadelphia: Mosby; 2010.)

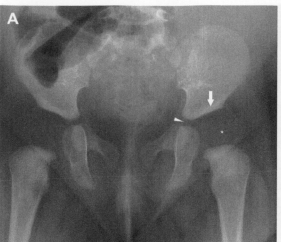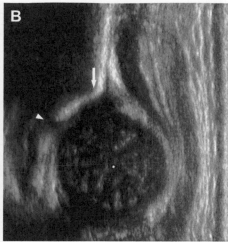

Fig. 3. Normal hip. (*A*) Anteroposterior radiograph of the pelvis and (*B*) coronal neutral view of the left hip ultrasound presented vertically. The osseous acetabular roof (*white arrow*) and the triradiate cartilage (*arrowhead*) are displayed on both images. The unossified femoral head (*white asterisk*) is covered by the acetabulum.

adequate penetration to the required depth, the medial aspect of the acetabulum. For newborns and infants up to 3 months of age, a 7.5 to 15 MHz transducer is usually sufficient. For large infants, from 3- to 6-months of age, a 5 MHz transducer might be required. Scanning is performed from a lateral and posterolateral approach in orthogonal coronal and transverse planes with respect to the pelvis. During scanning the infant should be relaxed. A quiet environment and a parent in contact with the infant (holding infant's arms) are helpful. The upper body can remain clothed. A well-fed infant, having been fed just prior to the examination, might also be more relaxed and cooperative. The examination can be performed with the baby in supine or decubitus position, or in between. Ambidextrous scanning is recommended to avoid cumbersome crossing of the examiner's hands. For a successful dynamic evaluation while scanning the right hip, the examiner holds the transducer in the left hand and the infant's leg in the right hand and the opposite for scanning the left hip. Two orthogonal planes relative to the pelvis, coronal and transverse, are obtained (**Figs. 1** and **2**). For teaching and orientation purposes, one notes that the coronal view scanning plane is similar to an anteroposterior radiograph (**Fig. 3**). However, because sonographic images are displayed with the transducer surface (footprint) at the top of the monitor, the orientation is lateral at the top and superior to left of the screen (**Fig. 4**). Likewise, transverse images are similar to axial cross-sectional imaging. Ultrasound images will display lateral at the top and anterior on the left or right of the screen (**Fig. 5**).

Coronal View

The coronal view is obtained from a lateral approach with the hip extended in neutral position (approximately 20 degrees of flexion) while the transducer is maintained in a coronal plane with respect to the acetabulum. The standard coronal plane includes three landmarks: (1) the iliac line, which is straight and parallel to the top margin of the image, (2) the transition point between the osseous iliac portion of the acetabulum and the triradiate cartilage, and (3) the echogenic lateral tip of the labrum extending laterally from the

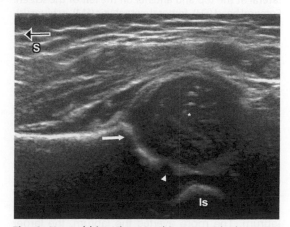

Fig. 4. Normal hip. Ultrasound image with the transducer surface (footprint) at the top of the image. The orientation is lateral at the top and superior to left of the screen (*black arrow*). Femoral head (*), osseous acetabular roof (*white arrow*), triradiate cartilage (*arrow head*) and ischium (Is). S, superior.

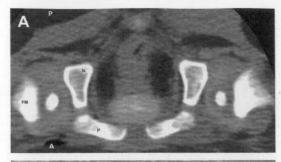

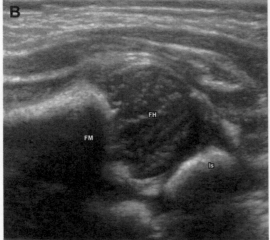

Fig. 5. Normal transverse view. (*A*) Axial CT image of the pelvis with patient in prone position, demonstrating the left femoral head with its ossified nucleus centered within the acetabulum. Black dots outlined the cartilaginous portion of the femoral head, pubis (p), anterior (A), posterior (P). If the image would be rotated approximately 40 degrees clockwise it will match the ultrasound transverse view. (*B*) Ultrasound of the left hip transverse view with the hip flexed. Ultrasound image displays lateral at the top and anterior on the left of the screen. Femoral head (FH), femoral metaphysic (FM), ischium (Is).

acetabulum (**Fig. 6**). The cartilaginous acetabular roof extends laterally over the femoral head. Hip morphology is assessed in this standard coronal view. The acetabular angle, α angle, is measured at the intersection of a horizontal line parallel to the lateral ilium and a line along the osseous acetabular roof. The α angle reflects the steepness of the osseous acetabular roof and relates to the coverage of the femoral head; greater than 60 degrees is considered normal (**Fig. 7**).[6,7,15]

Graf's method also describes a β angle that represents the elevation of the cartilaginous labrum. The more everted the labrum, the larger the β angle indicating subluxation or dislocation of the femur. Categorization of the hips according to Graf's method includes hip morphology and measurements for the α and β angles, and based on this technique, the hips are classified

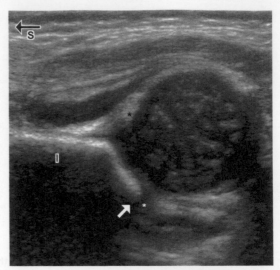

Fig. 6. Normal coronal view. Coronal neutral view with the transducer surface (footprint) at the top of the monitor, the orientation is lateral at the top and superior to left of the screen. Standard coronal plane on a 6-week-old baby demonstrates the iliac line (I) straight and parallel to the top margin of the image, the transition point between the osseous portion of the acetabulum (*white arrow*) and the triradiate cartilage (*white asterisk*) and the echogenic lateral tip of the labrum (*black asterisk*). S, superior.

into four main types and additional subtypes (**Table 1**).

Coronal images with the hip flexed to 90 degrees allows for a dynamic examination similar to the clinical examination with the Barlow[16] and Ortolani[17] tests. This image is also obtained

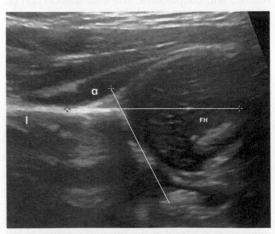

Fig. 7. Alpha angle. Coronal neutral view showing the acetabular angle (α angle), measured at the intersection of a horizontal line parallel to the lateral ilium (I) and a line along the osseous acetabular roof. FH, femoral head.

Table 1
Simplified synopsis of Graf sonographic hip types

Type	Description	Alpha Angle (Degrees)		Beta Angle Comment
I	Normal	>60	—	Should not dislocate in absence of a neuromuscular imbalance with altered biomechanics
IIa	Physiologic immature	50–59	—	—
—	—	<3 months of age	—	—
IIb	Delayed ossification	50–59	—	—
—	—	>3 months of age	—	—
IIc	Very deficient bony acetabulum but femoral head still concentric	43–49	<77	At this stage beta angle becomes important
D	Femoral head subluxed	43–49	>77	Increased beta angle signifies an elevated, everted labrum and subluxation
III	Dislocated	<43	>77	—
IV	Severe dysplasia/dislocation	Not measurable; flat, shallow, bony acetabulum	—	Labrum inverted; interposed between femoral head and ilium

From DiPietro MA, Harcke T. Pediatric musculoskeletal and spinal sonography. In: van Holsbeeck MT, Introcaso JH, editors. Musculoskeletal ultrasound. 2nd edition. St Louis (MO): Mosby; 2001. p. 277–323; and *Adapted from* Donaldson JS. Pediatric musculoskeletal US. In: Poznanski AK, Kirkpatrick JA Jr, editors. Diagnostic categorical course in pediatric radiology. Oak Brook (II): Radiological Society of North America Publications; 1989. p. 77–88; and Graf R. Guide to sonography of the infant hip. New York: Thieme Medical Publishers; 1987.

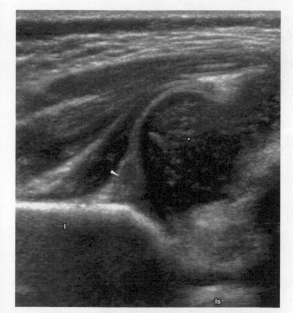

Fig. 8. Coronal view standard plane. In this 3-week-old infant with marked subluxation, the femoral head (*) is displaced superiorly and laterally and the acetabular cartilaginous roof is elevated (*arrowhead*). I, Ilium; Is, ischium.

through the mid-acetabulum similar to the coronal neutral view. If the femoral head is normally positioned, the relationship with the acetabulum will be maintained during the dynamic examination. Abduction and adduction of the femur, followed by adduction with posterior stress applied using a piston movement on the femur, comprises the dynamic stress portion of the study. This piston maneuver is essentially the Barlow test to evaluate instability. The femoral head migrates lateral and posteriorly with subluxation (**Fig. 8**), and the head is seen more posteriorly and superiorly with dislocation (**Fig. 9**). A subluxated or dislocated hip can be tested for reducibility by the clinical Ortolani maneuver, pulling the hip forward while abducting the flexed femur (**Fig. 10**).

Another technique was described by Morin, based on the coronal flexion view according to Harcke's method, to evaluate the percent coverage of the femoral head by the osseous acetabulum. Morin's technique was later modified by Terjesen,[18,19] and based on these measurements it was reported that all hips with more than 58% of the femoral head covered by the osseous acetabulum at ultrasound had normal radiographic acetabular angles, and those hips with less than 33% osseous coverage had a dysplastic acetabulum.[20]

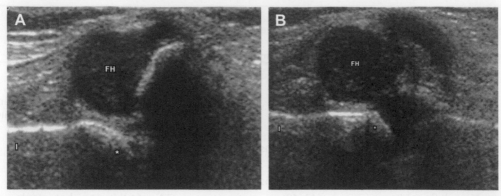

Fig. 9. Hip dislocation. (*A*) Coronal view on a 3-week-old infant demonstrates marked dislocation of the femoral head (FH) noted at the posterolateral aspect of the ilium (I). (*B*) Coronal image at the most posterior aspect of the acetabulum (*) showing the dislocated femoral head far posteriorly and laterally displaced.

Transverse View

Transverse scanning is performed from a postero-lateral approach with the transducer oriented in an axial plane with respect to the pelvis, and with the hip flexed 90 degrees. The ossified femoral meta-physis is seen anteriorly adjacent to the femoral head, and the osseous acetabulum is seen posterior to the femoral head. The posterior carti-laginous labrum is continuous with the osseous acetabulum. In this transverse view, the femoral metaphysis and the normal acetabulum produce a *u*-shaped configuration during abduction and a *v*-shaped configuration during adduction (**Fig. 11**). Dynamic evaluation is performed with

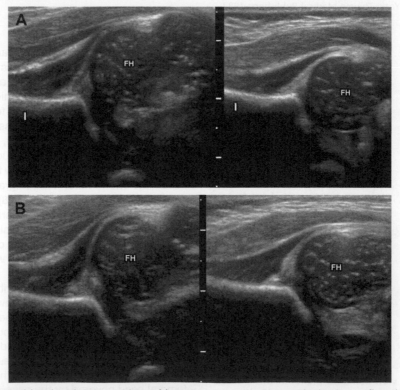

Fig. 10. Five-week-old girl with bilateral hip subluxation. Coronal views with the femur flexed 90 degrees. (*A*) Right hip. Markedly subluxated femoral head (FH), on dynamic examination during Ortolani maneuver the hip demonstrates reducibility. (*B*) Left hip. Markedly subluxated femoral head (FH), which can be partially reduced with abduction. Echogenic pulvinar is present in the acetabulum.

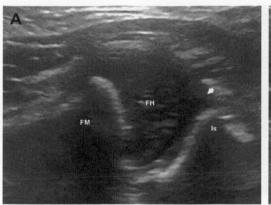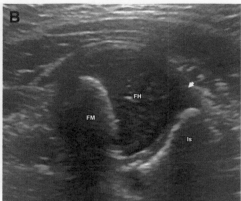

Fig. 11. Transverse flexion view. (*A*) Normal transverse ultrasound with abduction. The line of the femoral metaphysis (FM) and the bony portion of the ischium (Is) form a "U" configuration. (*B*) Normal transverse sonogram with adduction, now the lines of the femoral metaphysis and the ischium form a "V" configuration. FH, femoral head; cartilaginous acetabulum (*arrow*).

adduction and posterior stress similar to the clinical Barlow test. The subluxable femoral head will be displaced laterally relative to the acetabulum but will remain in contact with the ilium (**Fig. 12**). The dislocatable or dislocated femoral head will migrate more laterally and posteriorly or superiorly. A dislocated hip can be tested for reducibility by the clinical Ortolani maneuver, pulling the hip forward while abducting the flexed femur.

A transverse view with the hip in neutral position will demonstrate the femoral head placed against the acetabulum, centered at the triradiate cartilage (**Fig. 13**). In the subluxated hip, the femoral head remains in contact with the posterior acetabulum but soft-tissue echoes appear in a gap between the femoral head and the acetabulum. If dislocation is present, the femoral head will move posteriorly and superiorly, and bright echoes from the femoral shaft will obscure the acetabulum.

CLINICAL APPLICATION

Ultrasound of the hip may be obtained for diagnostic evaluation or management assessment. Diagnostic ultrasound is performed in newborns with risk factors for DDH or in newborns with abnormal hip findings on physical examination. When evaluating newborns it is important to consider the physiologic laxity and acetabular immaturity that normally can be seen in infants less than 4 weeks of age. Harcke and Grisssom[9] described physiologic laxity with stress as a normal variant at younger than 4 weeks, and Graf described a physiologically immature hip in infants younger than 3 months with delayed ossification as Type IIa.[7] Minor instability or acetabular immaturity tends to resolve spontaneously. Therefore, in a newborn with a risk factor and a normal physical examination, the best time to obtain a sonographic examination will be approximately 4- to 6-weeks of age so the transient laxity of physiologic immaturity could resolve and will not lead to multiple follow-up sonograms or to unnecessary treatment (**Fig. 14**). If the physical examination is abnormal, the ultrasound can be performed sooner, at 2- to 4-weeks of age.[1,3] Diagnostic assessment should include a complete ultrasound examination with coronal and transverse standard views. However,

Fig. 12. Femoral head subluxation. Transverse flexion view shows moderate posterolateral displacement of the subluxated femoral head (*). Hyperechoic material between the femoral head and the acetabulum represents a fibrofatty pulvinar. Cartilaginous acetabulum (*arrow*); FM, femoral metaphysis.

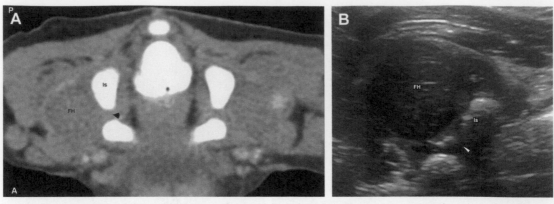

Fig. 13. Transverse view. (*A*) Axial CT image of the pelvis with patient in prone position, demonstrating the non-ossified femoral head (FH) centered within the acetabulum. If the image would be rotated approximately 40 degrees clockwise it will match the ultrasound transverse neutral view. (*B*) Transverse neutral view. The femoral head (FH) is centered within the acetabulum with the ischium (Is) posteriorly. Triradiate cartilage (*arrowhead*).

a four-view examination, including a coronal dynamic evaluation with the hip flexed to 90 degrees and a neutral transverse view, will provide additional assurance and the opportunity to confirm the morphologic and dynamic findings.

Hip ultrasound for DDH is highly specific and highly sensitive.[21–23] Variability of the stress applied and the degree of infant relaxation during the dynamic study introduces a subjective component. Lack of infant relaxation could hinder or prevent obtaining optimal stress views and produce a false-negative examination. Additionally, the acetabular anatomy may be obscured by patient body habitus or by a large femoral head ossification center in older infants (**Fig. 15**). Incorrect transducer positioning leads to false-positive cases. On the coronal view, incorrect transducer position in either the vertical, horizontal, or oblique plane will result in a coronal view out of the standard plane. Most commonly, the hip appears abnormal with an apparent steep roof and a shallow acetabulum (**Fig. 16**). On the transverse view, if the transducer is positioned lateral instead of posterolateral the hip may appear abnormal. The femoral shaft will obscure the acetabulum and the femoral head in patients with proximal femoral deficiency and coxa vara, or with arthrogryposis and hip contracture. In those cases, the cartilaginous greater trochanter may be inaccurately interpreted as a dislocated femoral head (**Fig. 17**).

Sonography is used periodically to assess DDH during treatment by splinting wherein the hips are held in a flexed and partially abducted position

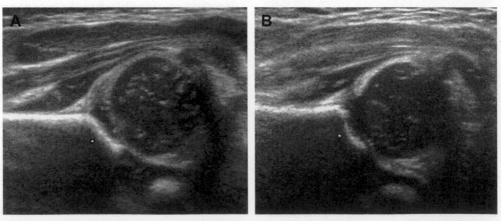

Fig. 14. Hip maturation. (*A*) Standard coronal plane view in a 2-week-old infant with mild acetabular immaturity with a slightly steep acetabulum (*). (*B*) Same patient 4 weeks later showing a mature acetabulum (*).

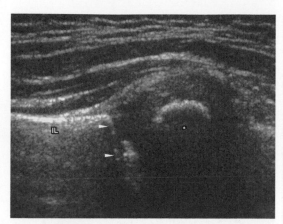

Fig. 15. Imaging the older infant. Standard coronal plane. Acetabular anatomy is obscured by femoral head ossification center (*) in an 11-month-old patient. The acetabular roof is partially visualized (*arrowheads*). IL, ilium.

over a period of weeks. The splint restricts adduction that would otherwise cause the lax hip to become subluxated or to dislocate. The commonly used Pavlik harness is a dynamic splint that allows a limited range of motion that keeps the hips partially flexed and abducted, maintaining the femoral head within the acetabulum, and thereby allowing the lax ligaments to tighten and the acetabulum to mature normally. Sequential non-stress ultrasounds are obtained while patients are in the harness to evaluate for appropriate location of the femoral head (**Fig. 18**). Therefore,

sonographic evaluation in the harness is focused on morphology and the dynamic examination is limited to no more than gentle abduction and adduction without stress maneuvers. Interval ultrasound evaluation in the harness can be performed weekly or every 2 or 3 weeks, depending on the severity of the dysplasia.

As ultrasound became recognized as a sensitive test for DDH, several approaches to define who should be screened were investigated. A study conducted by Rosendalh and colleagues in Norway evaluated three different screening models: clinical screening based exclusively on physical examination, general universal ultrasound of all infants, and selective ultrasound screening for high-risk patients. By performing selective screening ultrasound fewer cases were missed as compared with clinical screening. However, universal ultrasound screening did not produce a statistically significant advantage.[24] The applicability of current literature varies in different areas of the world. Although no statistically significant evidence has been shown, it is inferred from multiple well-designed observational studies that selective and universal ultrasounds reduce the number of late diagnosis of DDH.[25] In the United States, the American Academy of Pediatrics recommends repeated clinical examination by the pediatrician in every well-baby visit until 12 months of age. The examiner must understand that the Barlow/Ortolani test would become negative between 2 weeks and 2 months of age, with limited hip abduction being the key clinical sign of DDH. Once clinical signs are present, a confirmatory clinical examination performed by an orthopedic

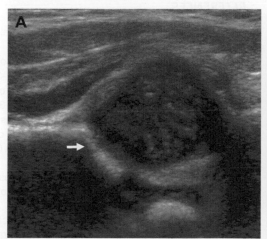
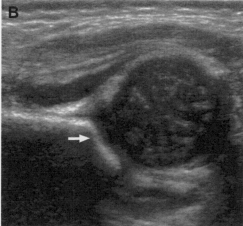

Fig. 16. Effect of poor positioning. Coronal views of the same patient. (*A*) Out of the standard plane, displaying a shallow acetabulum (*arrow*). (*B*) On coronal standard plane a normal acetabulum is evident.

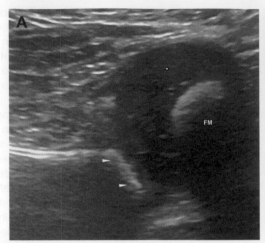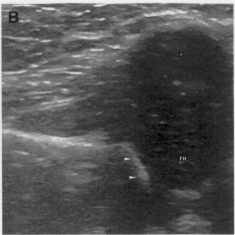

Fig. 17. Nine-week-old boy with hip contracture caused by arthrogryposis. (*A*) The unossified greater trochanter (*) may be mistaken as a lateral dislocated femoral head. The femoral metaphysis limits the visualization of the acetabulum and the femoral head. (*B*). During real-time scanning the unossified femoral head (FH) was seen within the acetabulum (*arrowheads*).

surgeon, sonographic examination, and radiographic examination will be secondary resources for the pediatrician to confirm the diagnosis. The ACR recommends ultrasound for infants with risk factors, including breech presentation or positive family history. Because of the increased bony development and the presence of the femoral head ossification nucleus by 4 months of age,

imaging generally shifts from ultrasound to radiography by 4- to 6- months of age.[26]

SUMMARY

Ultrasound is a safe, noninvasive, reliable, and reproducible method to evaluate for infant DDH that assesses hip morphology and hip stability. Once DDH has been diagnosed in the infant, sonography can be used to evaluate hip position and acetabular development during treatment. The optimal time and situation to screen for DDH continues to be studied and recommendations are revised. Meanwhile, it behooves the radiologist to perform and interpret hip sonography with attention to proper technique.

Fig. 18. Picture illustrating the position of the transducer to obtain a coronal view in a patient on a harness. (*From* DiPietro MA, Harcke T. Pediatric musculoskeletal and spinal sonography. In: van Holsbeeck MT, Introcaso JH, editors. Musculoskeletal ultrasound. 3rd edition. Philadelphia: Mosby; 2010.)

REFERENCES

1. DiPietro MA, Harcke T. Pediatric musculoskeletal and spinal sonography. In: van Holsbeeck MT, Introcaso JH, editors. Musculoskeletal ultrasound. 2nd edition. St Louis (MO): Mosby; 2001. p. 277–323.
2. Lee MC, Eberson CP. Growth and development of the child's hip. Orthop Clin North Am 2006;37:119–32.
3. DiPietro MA, Harcke T. Developmental dysplasia of the hip. In: Slovis TL, editor. Caffeys's pediatric diagnostic imaging, vol 2. 11th edition. Philadelphia (PA): Mosby Elsevier; 2008. p. 3049–67.
4. Place MJ, Parkin DM, Fitton JM. Effectiveness of neonatal screening for congenital dislocation of the hip. Lancet 1978;2:249–51.
5. Harcke HT, Lee MS, Sinning L, et al. Ossification center of the infant hip: sonographic and radiographic correlation. AJR Am J Roentgenol 1986; 147:317–21.

6. Graf R. The diagnosis of congenital hip-joint dislocation by the ultrasonic compound treatment. Arch Orthop Trauma Surg 1980;97:117–33.

7. Graf R. Classification of hip joint dysplasia by means of sonography. Arch Orthop Trauma Surg 1984;102:248–55.

8. Harcke HT, Clarke NMP, Lee MS, et al. Examination of the infant hip with real-time ultrasonography. J Ultrasound Med 1984;3:131–7.

9. Harcke HT, Grissom LE. Performing dynamic sonography of the infant hip. AJR Am J Roentgenol 1990;155:837–44.

10. Harcke HT, Graf R, Clarke NMP. Consensus meeting on hip sonography. Alfred I. duPont Institute. Wilmington (DE), September 23–24, 1993.

11. Harcke HT, Grissom LE. Infant hip sonography: current concepts. Semin Ultrasound CT MR 1994;15:256–63.

12. American College of Radiology. ACR appropriateness criteria. ® Pediatric imaging. Developmental dysplasia of the hip. Available at: www.acr.org.

13. American College of Radiology. ACR practice guideline for the performance of ultrasound examination for detection and assessment of developmental dysplasia of the hip. American College of Radiology. Available at: www.acr.org [Standards].

14. American Institute of Ultrasound in Medicine. AIUM practice guideline for the performance of an ultrasound examination for detection and assessment of developmental dysplasia of the hip. J Ultrasound Med. 2009;28:114–9.

15. Wientroub S, Grill F. Current concepts review Ultrasonography in Developmental dysplasia of the hip. J Bone Joint Surg 2000;82A(7):1004–18.

16. Barlow TG. Early diagnosis and treatment of the congenital dislocation of the hip. J Bone Joint Surg Br 1962;44B:292–301.

17. Ortolani M. The classic: congenital hip dysplasia in the light of early and very early diagnosis. Clin Orthop 1976;119:6–10.

18. Morin C, Harcke HT, MacEwen GD. The infant hip: Real-time US assessment of acetabular development. Radiology 1985;157:673–7.

19. Terjesen T, Bredland T, Berg V. Ultrasound for hip assessment in the newborn. J Bone Joint Surg Br 1989;71:767–73.

20. Terjesen T, Holen KJ, Tegnander. Hip abnormalities detected by ultrasound in clinically normal newborn infants. J Bone Joint Surg 1996;78B:636–40.

21. Clarke NMP, Harcke HT, McHugh P, et al. Real-time ultrasound in the diagnosis of congenital dislocation and dysplasia of the hip. J Bone Joint Surg 1985;67B:406–12.

22. Berman L, Klenerman L. Ultrasound screening for hip abnormalities: preliminary findings in 1001 neonates. Br Med J 1986;293:719–22.

23. Tonnis D, Storch K, Ulbrich H. Results of newborn screening for CDH with and without sonography and correlation of risk factors. J Pediatr Orthop 1990;10:145–52.

24. Rosendahl K, Markestad T, Terje Lie R. Ultrasound screening for developmental dysplasia of the hip in the neonate: the effect on treatment rate and prevalence of late cases. Pediatrics 1994;94:47–52.

25. Rosendahl K, Toma P. Ultrasound in the diagnosis of developmental dysplasia of the hip in newborns. The European approach. A review of methods, accuracy and clinical validity. Eur Radiol 2007;17:1960–7.

26. Karmazyn BK, Gunderman RB, Coley BD, et al. ACR Appropriateness criteria on developmental dysplasia of the hip-child. J Am Coll Radiol 2009;6:551–7.

Pediatric Musculoskeletal Ultrasound

Oscar M. Navarro, MD[a,b,*], Dimitri A. Parra, MD[a,c]

KEYWORDS

• Musculoskeletal • Ultrasound • Children

Ultrasonography (US) is a valuable tool in the diagnosis, follow-up, and treatment of the conditions that may affect the musculoskeletal system in the pediatric population. Apart from the well-known advantages of US (low cost, lack of radiation, and widespread availability), the inherent features of the immature skeleton widen the diagnostic capabilities of this modality. The nonossified portions of the bones and the lack of thick adipose tissue planes in children provide an excellent window for assessment of joints, cartilage, tendons, and muscles.[1,2] US also plays a significant role in the diagnosis of soft tissue tumors and inflammatory processes and in guiding joint interventions and soft tissue biopsies. Magnetic resonance (MR) imaging also plays a major role in the diagnosis of musculoskeletal conditions.[2] Therefore, in an effective and well-organized pediatric radiology department both modalities should be used in a complementary fashion. Because of the high yield of US, in many instances it is the first and only modality used for diagnosis. However, a rational use of US and MR imaging requires a thorough understanding of the strengths and weaknesses of both.

Although there are many well-established applications of US in pediatric musculoskeletal disease and many more potential applications, the objective of this article is to review those that are more commonly seen in the daily practice, including musculoskeletal inflammatory processes, noninfectious articular pathology, and soft tissue tumors.

TECHNIQUE

The use of high frequency linear array transducers is indispensable in the evaluation of musculoskeletal pathology because of the high-detailed images provided by these probes. Sector-array transducers of lower frequency may be required for the assessment of joints such as hip and shoulder and the evaluation of deeply located soft tissue lesions, particularly in older children. Color and spectral Doppler interrogation are particularly useful especially in cases of soft tissue tumor and soft tissue/joint inflammation.

The examination must be done in a quiet room using warm gel and if possible with the child accompanied by his or her parents or guardians. In infants, the examination can be easily performed with the child in the parent's arms. Sedation is almost never needed for diagnostic US; however, sedation or general anesthesia is warranted for US-guided interventions. A detailed clinical history and information provided by the parents in combination with review of any pertinent previous imaging studies are helpful and often crucial for obtaining high-yield examinations.

NORMAL SONOGRAPHIC MUSCULOSKELETAL ANATOMY

To recognize pathologic processes affecting the musculoskeletal system, the pediatric radiologist must be aware of the normal anatomy and normal

a Department of Medical Imaging, University of Toronto, Canada
b Department of Diagnostic Imaging, The Hospital for Sick Children, 555 University Avenue, Toronto, Ontario M5G 1X8, Canada
c Division of Image Guided Therapy, Department of Diagnostic Imaging, The Hospital for Sick Children, Toronto, Ontario M5G 1X8, Canada
* Corresponding author. Department of Diagnostic Imaging, The Hospital for Sick Children, 555 University Avenue, Toronto, Ontario M5G 1X8, Canada.
E-mail address: oscar.navarro@sickkids.ca (O.M. Navarro).

Ultrasound Clin 4 (2009) 457–470
doi:10.1016/j.cult.2009.10.003

US appearance of soft tissues and joints. The dermis and epidermis are seen as an echogenic thin layer superficial to the hypoechoic subcutaneous tissue (hypodermis). Some thin echogenic tracts of connective tissue can normally be seen crossing the hypodermis. The muscular fascia appears as a thin echogenic layer superficial to the muscle planes.[3] Muscles have a highly organized cytoarchitecture with multiple linear fibrous septa on a hypoechoic background (muscular parenchyma).[4] Tendons appear as echogenic fibrillar structures with multiple parallel lines in the longitudinal plane and multiple "dotlike" echoes in the transverse plane. The synovial sheath is seen as a thin, fluid-containing structure that surrounds the echogenic tendon fiber.[5,6] Tendons and muscles should be examined with an angle of insonation perpendicular to their long axis because their reflectivity is angle-dependent (anisotropy). Anisotropy may cause artifact and mimic abnormalities in these structures, which can be avoided with the use of beam angulation.[7]

Within the joints and in nonossified bones, cartilage appears as a homogeneous hypoanechoic layer limited by thin, sharp, and slightly hyperechoic margins. Normal articular cartilage is homogeneous with a sharp interface with the joint space and a sharp interface with the adjacent hyperechoic bone.[6] The joint cavities and articular capsules are barely seen or invisible with US in normal conditions. A small amount of anechoic joint fluid can be seen in healthy individuals.[6] Ligaments are seen as echogenic fibrillar structures.[5] Peripheral nerves are seen as hypoechoic fascicles surrounded by a thin echogenic layer (perineurium and epineurium).[8]

MUSCULOSKELETAL INFECTIONS

Musculoskeletal infections are of common occurrence in children and may affect the bones, joints, and soft tissues. Imaging is often required in the moderate and severe cases and in some particular patients such as those in immunosuppression. US may be useful in the differentiation of infectious processes from other conditions (particularly tumors), in the determination of site and extent of involvement, in the search of a drainable abscess formation, in the identification of a foreign body, and to provide guidance for diagnostic or therapeutic intervention (aspiration, drainage, or biopsy).[9]

Cellulitis

Cellulitis, an infectious inflammatory involvement of the skin and subcutaneous tissues, is often diagnosed clinically although occasionally it may present clinically as a soft tissue mass. US is often requested to exclude the presence of an abscess associated with cellulitis. In cellulitis, there is increased echogenicity and thickening of the subcutaneous fat with gradual transition from abnormal to normal echogenicity that may progress to a cobblestone appearance caused by development of hypoechoic strands between the hyperechoic fatty lobules.[9,10]

Abscess

Abscess is a focal suppurative collection, which in the soft tissues usually represents a complication of an infectious process such as cellulitis, subperiosteal abscess, pyomyositis, and lymphadenitis. The US appearance is highly variable although more typically an abscess appears as a hypoechoic fluid collection surrounded by increased echogenicity of the adjacent soft tissues. The diagnosis can be difficult if the abscess is hyperechoic or isoechoic to adjacent soft tissues, in which cases gentle pressure with the transducer may elicit the motion of particles within the collection, indicating its fluid nature.[10] Doppler US characteristically reveals peripheral hyperemia and absence of flow within the contents of the abscess.

Soft Tissue Foreign Body

Although radiography is often used as the primary imaging modality for detection of foreign bodies in the soft tissues, US offers several advantages compared with radiography. US allows detection of radioopaque and radiolucent foreign bodies, the latter being more frequent than the former. US also allows easy depiction of the relationship of the foreign body to adjacent structures and can be used in real time for guidance of foreign body removal.[11]

On US, a foreign body appears as a hyperechoic structure, which in case of metal or glass (large radius of curvature or smooth surface) has dirty shadowing and posterior reverberation artifact. In case of wooden fragments (small radius of curvature or rough surface), there is clean posterior acoustic shadow without reverberation artifact.[11] Associated inflammatory reaction with granulation tissue, edema, or hemorrhage often develops after 24 hours, appearing on US as a hypoechoic halo surrounding and increasing the conspicuity of the foreign body (**Fig. 1**).

Pyomyositis

Pyomyositis is a primary suppurative infection of striated muscle, much more frequently seen in tropical regions, and although rare in temperate climates its incidence is increasing, particularly in

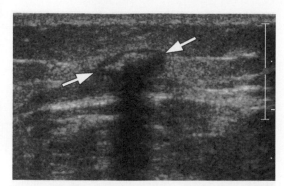

Fig. 1. Wooden foreign body in a 13-year-old boy. Transverse US image of the right lower leg shows within the subcutaneous tissues the presence of a well-defined hyperechoic structure (*arrows*) that casts acoustic shadow without reverberation artifact. A thin hypoechoic halo representing associated inflammatory response is also evident.

immunocompromised patients (eg, those with human immunodeficiency virus infection, varicella, or malnutrition, or undergoing chemotherapy). Additional risk factors include trauma, diabetes mellitus, chronic steroid use, and connective tissue disorders.[10,12] The most common etiologic agent is *Staphylococcus aureus*. It usually affects buttocks and thighs, more commonly with focal involvement of a single muscle, although multifocal involvement is not rare. The clinical diagnosis is usually challenging as the symptoms of myalgias, general malaise, and fever are nonspecific, and children have more difficulty in localizing the pain.

Three clinical stages have been described. In stage I (initial-invasive), phlegmonous changes are evident on US, with muscle edema, distortion of the fibrillar pattern of the muscles and ill-defined areas of decreased echogenicity. In stage II (suppurative-purulent), there is abscess formation. Stage III (late) is associated with severe toxicity and there may be extension of the infection into the adjacent bone and joint space.[10,12]

Osteomyelitis

Osteomyelitis represents infection of the bone and bone marrow. In children, it is more frequently of bacterial cause, usually *Staphylococcus aureus*. Pediatric osteomyelitis is often hematogenous in origin and usually begins in the metaphysis of long bones and metaphyseal equivalents. In infants and after the closure of the growth plates, because of continuity of the metaphyseal vascularity with the epiphysis, there may be extension of the infection into the epiphysis and eventually into the articular space. With progression of the infection, the increased pressure within the medullary cavity

allows extension of the infection to the cortex, subperiosteal space and adjacent soft tissues. Therefore, abscesses can develop in the medullary cavity, subperiosteal space, and soft tissues.[12]

The radiographic changes of osteomyelitis may not be visible until 7 to 10 days after the onset of the infection. For this reason, some investigators have advocated the use of US, which can identify changes before they become apparent on radiography.[10] These US changes include deep edema, periosteal thickening, intraarticular fluid collection, and subperiosteal abscess formation (**Fig. 2**), the latter defined by elevation of the periosteum greater than 2 mm.[10] Cortical erosion can also become evident on US.[9]

With the increased availability of MR imaging, the role of US in the evaluation of osteomyelitis is now probably secondary. However, in the US evaluation of patients with a soft tissue infection the adjacent bone should also be assessed to look for changes suggestive of osteomyelitis that may not be clinically suspected.

Infectious Arthritis

The presence of joint swelling, pain, and increased temperature in a child is a medical emergency. The differential diagnosis is broad, but the most significant cause for such presentation is septic arthritis, which if untreated may result in joint destruction, limited functionality, and deformity[13]; its mortality has been described to be as high as 10%.[14] Infection can reach the joint by hematogenous spread,

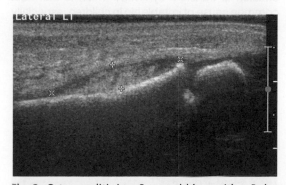

Fig. 2. Osteomyelitis in a 2-year-old boy with a 3-day history of erythematous swelling in the lateral aspect of left lower leg, inability to weight-bear and fever. Longitudinal US image of the inferior aspect of the left fibula shows an echogenic subperiosteal fluid collection (*between cursors*), compatible with an abscess, associated with scalloping and irregularity of the underlying cortex in the distal diametaphyseal region. There is swelling and increased echogenicity of the overlying soft tissues in keeping with cellulitis. Blood cultures were positive for group A *Streptococcus*.

direct contamination, or indirect contamination from a nearby infection.[15] In neonates, the most common organism is *Staphylococcus aureus*. Other potential pathogens are *Escherichia coli*, group B streptococci, other gram-negatives, and *Candida albicans*. In older children *Staphylococcus aureus* and group A streptococci are the organisms most commonly encountered. *Neisseria gonorrhoeae* can be seen in adolescents, *Salmonella* in patients with sickle cell disease, and fungal, parasitic, and mycobacterial infections in immunocompromised patients.[15]

In a patient with clinical signs of infection, the most important US finding suggestive of septic arthritis is joint effusion, which is usually seen at an early stage of the disease. This fluid can be hypoechoic and clearly demarcated from the joint structures (**Fig. 3**) or hyperechoic and less clearly demarcated from the synovium or capsule (**Fig. 4**).[9] Increased Doppler flow and synovial thickening can also be seen in the joint.[9] None of the US characteristics of the joint effusion allow the radiologist to conclude that the fluid is infected or not.[16] Absence of joint effusion in septic arthritis is extremely rare[16]; however, in joints with nondistensible capsules, the absence of fluid does not exclude infection and further imaging/interventions should be performed if the clinical suspicion is persistent.[9]

Of special mention is the differential diagnosis of septic arthritis of the hip. If septic arthritis or other noninfectious causes of arthritis are excluded, the most likely diagnosis in the presence of hip joint effusion is transient synovitis, which is the most common cause of irritable hip in children, especially between the ages of 3 and 8 years.[13] Transient

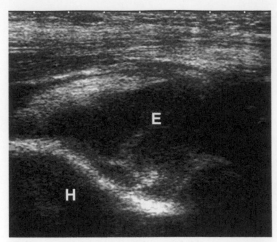

Fig. 4. Septic arthritis of the right elbow in a 10-year-old girl who presented with a 5-day history of fever and elbow pain. Longitudinal US image of the posterior recess of the right elbow show a moderate to large-sized echogenic joint effusion (E) that is difficult to differentiate from the joint capsule. A surgical lavage was performed. H, humerus.

synovitis is a benign, idiopathic, self-limited inflammation of the synovial lining. US features, which are bilateral in one-fourth of cases, may include joint effusion and synovial thickening (**Fig. 5**).[16]

US is suited for image-guided needle aspiration of joint effusion in suspected cases of septic arthritis, allowing early diagnosis and onset of treatment, which in turn decreases the chances of permanent sequelae.

NONINFECTIOUS ARTHROPATHIES
Juvenile Idiopathic Arthritis

Juvenile idiopathic arthritis (JIA) is the most common chronic rheumatic disease in childhood, involving a group of disorders characterized by chronic arthritis.[17,18] Its incidence ranges from 1 to 22 per 100,000.[17] JIA is defined as persistent arthritis for more than 6 weeks with an onset at less than 16 years of age, after excluding other causes of joint inflammation.[19] The cause of JIA seems to be multifactorial, and may be related to genetic factors associated with triggering events such as psychological stress, abnormal hormone levels, trauma, or infections.[17] The histopathology of the inflamed joints shows infiltration by lymphocytes, plasma cells, macrophages, and dendritic cells associated with a proliferation of fibroblasts and macrophages.[20] The classification of arthritis in children has been challenging, with that developed by the International League of Associations for Rheumatology (ILAR) in the 1990s being the most common in use.[17,20] In this classification,

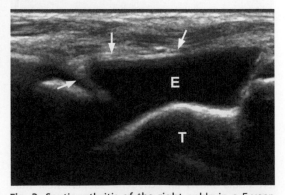

Fig. 3. Septic arthritis of the right ankle in a 5-year-old boy with history of cellulitis of unknown origin and ankle pain. Longitudinal US image of the anterior ankle recess shows a moderate-sized hypoechoic joint effusion (E), well demarcated from the thickened synovial capsule (*arrows*). The diagnosis was confirmed at surgery. T, talus.

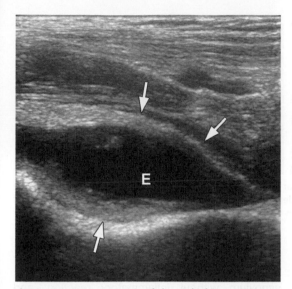

Fig. 5. Transient synovitis of the right hip in a 6-year-old boy with a 2-day history of hip pain and limping. Longitudinal US image shows a moderate-sized hypoechoic hip joint effusion (E) associated with thickening of the capsule (*arrows*). Septic arthritis was excluded and was managed as a transient synovitis of the hip. There was complete recovery with no sequelae.

JIA includes 7 subtypes of arthritis according to the clinical features during the first 6 months of disease and with the following frequencies: oligoarticular JIA (50%–60%), polyarticular JIA (rheumatoid factor positive and negative) (30%–35%), systemic JIA (10%–20%), juvenile psoriatic arthritis (2%–15%), enthesitis-related arthritis (1%–7%), and undifferentiated arthritis.[17] The knee joint is the most commonly involved joint in JIA (77%), followed by the ankle (58%)[21]; however, many other joints can be affected and become symptomatic, including those in the hands, wrists, feet, hips, and temporomandibular joints.

In the acute setting of joint swelling, US can identify joint effusion, synovial thickening (**Fig. 6**), and synovial cysts. Signs of inflammation on US include thickening, nodularity, and hyperechogenicity of the synovium around the joint space. The increase in size and distribution of the synovium usually means increase of the disease activity, whereas a decrease of the joint effusion suggests improvement.[22] Color Doppler US can confirm the synovial proliferation and also assess the degree of vascularity and activity of the inflammation. Cartilage proliferation and erosions can be seen in late stages of the disease.[22]

Tenosynovitis is another manifestation of JIA, which in some patients can explain absence of response to treatment when only the joints are injected. Tenosynovitis is found in up to 71% of JIA patients with symptomatic ankles, the medial compartment being the most frequently involved.[23] Increase of fluid within the synovial sheath (**Fig. 7**), hyperemia, and sheath thickening (**Fig. 8**) are the most characteristic US features of tenosynovitis.[6]

US is a valuable tool for image-guided steroid injections into joints that are not accessible by anatomic landmarks and for tendon sheaths in which the space for injection is limited.

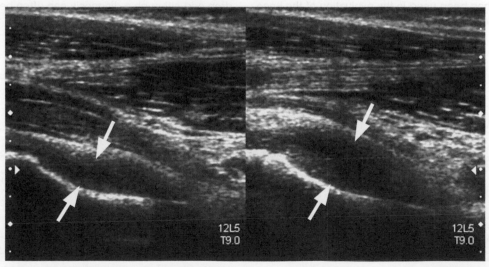

Fig. 6. Bilateral hip involvement in an 11-year-old girl, diagnosed with JIA at 4 years of age, who presented with acute onset of bilateral hip pain. Longitudinal US images of both hips show bilateral hip joint effusion (*arrows*), moderate-sized on the right and small on the left, compatible with arthritis secondary to JIA. The symptoms responded to medical therapy.

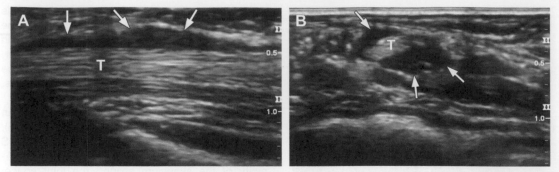

Fig. 7. Tenosynovitis in a 5-year-old girl with oligoarticular JIA and wrist pain. (*A*) Longitudinal and (*B*) transverse US images of the palmar aspect of the wrist show a moderate amount of fluid (*arrows*) in the tendon sheath of the right flexor carpi ulnaris tendon (T), compatible with tenosynovitis.

Hemophilia

Hemophilia is an X-linked recessive disorder characterized by a deficiency of clotting factors VIII or IX. Its pathogenesis is not well understood and it has an incidence of approximately 1 in 10,000 to 1 in 30,000 live male births.[24] Joints are the most frequent sites of bleeding, which occurs most frequently in knees, elbows, and ankles (**Fig. 9**).[25] Hemophilic joint disease secondary to recurrent hemarthrosis is one of the most disabling and expensive complications of hemophilia.[24] The episodes of hemarthrosis during childhood result in synovitis, synovial proliferation, increased vascularity, and chronic inflammation (**Fig. 10**). With time there is pannus formation and destructive arthritis (narrowing of joint space, subchondral bone irregularity, osteoporosis, joint surface incongruity, limitation of motion).[24,25]

US has been used in the evaluation of the knee in children with hemophilia. In patients without radiological changes, US may reveal a slight increase of joint fluid, a moderately hypertrophic synovium without inflammatory reaction, and normal cartilage. In patients with mild to moderate radiological changes, US may show significant hypertrophy and hyperemia of the synovium associated with mild to moderate joint effusion (**Fig. 10**). In children with advanced disease, US may show significant synovial hypertrophy with a mild inflammatory reaction, a normal amount of fluid, joint deformity, and muscle atrophy.[25] Cartilage damage can also be seen with US and correlates well with the degree of joint involvement seen on radiography.[25]

SOFT TISSUE MASSES

Soft tissue masses are a common finding in children and although a diagnosis can often be made on clinical grounds, in many instances further

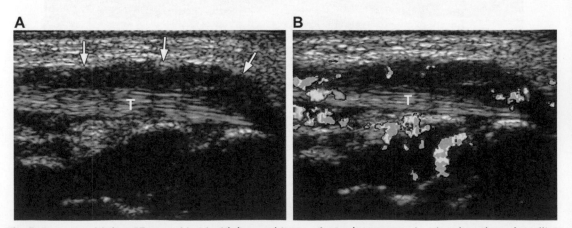

Fig. 8. Tenosynovitis in a 17-year-old girl with known history of JIA who presented with wrist pain and swelling. (*A*) Longitudinal gray scale and (*B*) longitudinal color Doppler US images of the dorsal aspect of the wrist show thickening in (*A*) (*arrows*) and hyperemia in (*B*) of the sheath of the extensor carpi radialis longus tendon (T), compatible with tenosynovitis.

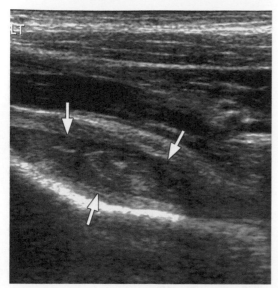

Fig. 9. Hemarthrosis in a 10-year-old boy with hemophilia B who had a history of a fall while skiing with a superficial knee bleed treated with factor IX. Four days later he presented with left anterior thigh pain. Longitudinal US image of the left hip show a moderate-sized echogenic joint effusion (*arrows*) compatible with hemarthrosis.

imaging evaluation is required to establish if a soft tissue mass is truly present, to confirm a presumed clinical diagnosis, to assess deeper extension, or to determine relationship to adjacent anatomic

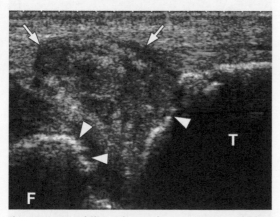

Fig. 10. Hemophilic arthropathy in a 17-year-old boy with repetitive episodes of knee hemarthrosis. Longitudinal US image of the anterolateral aspect of the left knee shows a heterogeneous mass with hypoechoic and hyperechoic areas extending from the joint space into the more superficial soft tissues (*arrows*) caused by a combination of hemarthrosis, synovial thickening, and hemosiderin deposition. There is also irregularity (*arrowheads*) of the adjacent cortical surfaces of the distal femur (F) and proximal tibia (T) caused by erosive changes. (*Courtesy of* Arun Mohanta, MBBS, Toronto, Canada.)

structures. US is particularly helpful in the evaluation of small and superficial lesions by assessing shape, volume, margins, compressibility, and vascularity and by allowing differentiation between cystic and solid tumors. MR imaging is usually required for larger and deeper lesions.

Most soft tissue masses in children are benign and of these the most common are vascular lesions, which are discussed elsewhere in this issue. The remaining causes of soft tissue masses are varied, with the most common being fibrous and fibrohistiocytic tumors and pseudotumors.[26] Malignant masses are rare in children; they do not exhibit specific US features that allow differentiation from benign masses and therefore require histologic diagnosis. For a more detailed review of the current classification of soft tissue tumors, the reader is encouraged to consult the World Health Organization classification of such lesions.[27]

Because of the broad spectrum of soft tissue masses and often nonspecific US appearance, this section reviews only those that are more prevalent in childhood and those in which US is helpful in establishing a specific diagnosis. However, a specific diagnosis can only rarely be made from US findings alone, practically always requiring correlation with findings on the physical examination (body site affected, changes in the overlying skin, tenderness, features on palpation) and clinical history (patient's age, duration, pattern of growth, systemic symptoms, predisposing conditions).

Fibrous Tumors

Fibrous tumors are mesenchymal tumors with fibroblastic and myofibroblastic features. The most common in children are nodular fasciitis, myositis ossificans, fibrous hamartoma of infancy, myofibroma/myofibromatosis, fibromatosis colli, fibroma of tendon sheath, deep or desmoid-type fibromatosis, superficial fibromatosis, and fibrolipomatosis.

Nodular fasciitis is an idiopathic, benign, localized tumor usually of the subcutaneous tissues that may present clinically as a rapidly growing lesion, although it rarely exceeds 4 cm. Intramuscular and intermuscular locations have also been reported. It is commonly seen in the upper extremities, particularly the volar aspect of the forearm, but may also affect the lower extremities, trunk, and head and neck.[28] On US, nodular fasciitis usually appears as a well-defined hypoechoic nodular or ovoid subcutaneous lesion, often based on the superficial fascia of the underlying muscles, of low or mixed echogenicity, with peripheral and central flow on Doppler evaluation (**Fig. 11**).[28]

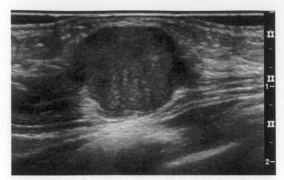

Fig. 11. Nodular fasciitis in a 2-year-old girl who presented with a 1-day history of a firm, tender mass in the chest wall. Transverse US image of the right chest wall shows a well-defined, homogeneous, hypoechoic nodular mass involving the pectoralis muscle and overlying subcutaneous tissues. The diagnosis was confirmed on histology.

Fibromatosis colli is an entity in which US can establish a specific diagnosis although the diagnosis is often made clinically. Fibromatosis colli is a fibrous reaction to injury of the sternocleidomastoid muscle believed to be related to venous occlusion secondary to intrauterine malposition or prolonged labor.[29] The child may present with torticollis or a neck mass commonly 2 to 8 weeks after birth. On US, fibromatosis colli may present as fusiform enlargement of the sternocleidomastoid muscle or as a focal mass, which can be hyperechoic, of mixed echogenicity, or hypoechoic, usually with increased vascularity on color Doppler interrogation (**Fig. 12**).[29,30] There is no abnormality of the adjacent soft tissues.

Myofibromatosis is the most common fibrous tumor of infancy, occurring mainly in infants less than 2 years old; more than half of the infants are diagnosed at birth.[31,32] It may present as solitary (myofibroma) or as multicentric masses (myofibromatosis). These tumors often have a good prognosis as they show spontaneous regression in 1 to 2 years after presentation, although some of the multicentric myofibromatosis are associated with poor outcome, particularly those with significant visceral involvement. Two histologic patterns have been described, one of which shows vessels arranged in a pattern that resembles hemangiopericytoma, and, therefore, it is believed that the infantile hemangiopericytoma is part of the spectrum of myofibromas rather than a separate entity.[27] Myofibromas have a variable US appearance. Koujok and colleagues[33] describe most lesions having an anechoic center with little flow, although in some cases the lesions have a more homogeneous solid appearance with occasional calcifications (**Fig. 13**).

Desmoid-type or deep fibromatosis is also a benign fibroblastic/myofibroblastic tumor but one that tends to show a more infiltrative growth pattern with a tendency to local recurrence, hence its label of aggressive fibromatosis.[34] Familial adenomatous polyposis and Gardner syndrome are predisposing conditions for the formation of

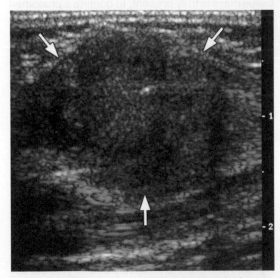

Fig. 13. Myofibromatosis in 5-week-old girl who presented with a 3-week history of hard lump in the right upper arm and 2 nodules in the left lower leg. Longitudinal US image of the right upper arm shows a well-defined hypoechoic nodule involving the muscles and subcutaneous tissues (*arrows*). A small hyperechoic focus seen centrally within the lesion represents calcification. The diagnosis was confirmed on histology. Further investigation demonstrated also involvement of pelvic viscera, left kidney, bones, and lungs, in keeping with multicentric myofibromatosis.

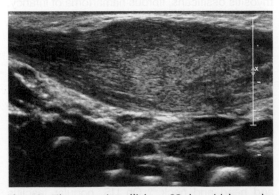

Fig. 12. Fibromatosis colli in a 23-day-old boy who presented with a left-sided neck mass. Longitudinal US image shows fusiform enlargement of the sternocleidomastoid muscle. Within the expanded muscle a large area of increased echogenicity with loss of the normal fibrillar pattern is identified.

these tumors, although they are more often sporadic. In children, this type of fibromatosis is more often seen in the first decade and more frequently involves the musculature of the trunk and extremities.[35] There is little in the literature regarding US appearances of desmoid-type fibromatosis. In the authors' experience, desmoid fibromatosis tends to have a nonspecific appearance on US (**Fig. 14**), although a spindle shape of the mass has been described in intramuscular lesions and the presence of intralesional hyperechoic areas and a fibrillar pattern have also been described as common features.[36]

Adipocytic Tumors

Adipocytic tumors are tumors derived from mature or precursor adipocytic cells, and include lipoma, lipoblastoma, and liposarcoma. The presence of fat is not exclusive of adipocytic neoplasms as fat can also be demonstrated in fibrous tumors (fibrous hamartoma of infancy, fibrolipomatosis) and in involuting hemangiomas of infancy. On the other hand, some forms of liposarcoma may not contain any recognizable mature fat at all.

Lipomas, which are benign tumors comprised of mature adipocytes, account for about two-thirds of adipocytic tumors in children.[37] They are more frequently found in the upper back, neck, proximal extremities, and abdomen. They are more often superficial, involving the subcutaneous tissues, although deep lipomas involving the musculature are not uncommon. The US features are variable, being described as hyperechoic, hypoechoic, or isoechoic to muscle and of mixed echogenicity, and can be of well-defined or ill-defined borders.[38] The presentation of lipomas as an elliptical mass

with a parallel orientation in relation to the skin surface (**Fig. 15**), hyperechoic compared with adjacent muscle, and containing hyperechoic lines perpendicular to the ultrasound beam has been considered characteristic by some investigators.[39] Absence of vascularity is often demonstrated on color Doppler interrogation.

Lipoblastomas are also benign tumors and account for about 30% of adipocytic tumors.[37] They can be found in any site where embryonal fatty tissue is present, although they are more commonly seen in the subcutaneous tissues of the extremities and trunk.[37] In contrast to lipomas, these are rapidly growing tumors and are usually diagnosed in children less than 3 years of age. On US, lipoblastomas usually appear as masses of homogeneous and increased echogenicity (**Fig. 16**), although mixed echogenicity and fluid-filled spaces have also been reported.[40]

Liposarcomas are rare in children, and the myxoid type is more frequently seen in this age group. They more often present in the deep soft tissues of the lower extremities. The US features are nonspecific.

Peripheral Nerve Sheath Tumors

Although not strictly originating in the musculoskeletal system, tumors of the peripheral nerves may present as soft tissue masses. These tumors include the benign schwannoma (also known as

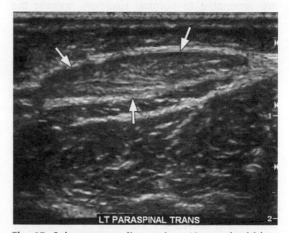

Fig. 15. Subcutaneous lipoma in a 12-month-old boy who presented with a 2-month history of nontender nodule in the left paraspinal region of the back, which has not shown noticeable growth since first noticed. Transverse US image shows a well-defined, elliptical mass (*arrows*) in the subcutaneous tissues of the left paraspinal region with a parallel orientation to the skin surface. The mass is slightly hyperechoic compared with the normal subcutaneous tissues and muscles. The diagnosis was confirmed on histology.

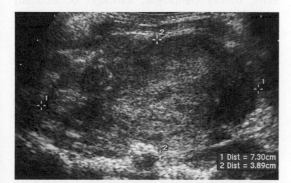

Fig. 14. Desmoid-type, deep or aggressive fibromatosis in a 14-year-old girl who presented with a 2-week history of rapidly growing, nontender left cervical mass. Longitudinal US image shows a large, solid heterogeneous mass (*between cursors*) deep to the left sternocleidomastoid muscle. The diagnosis was confirmed on histology.

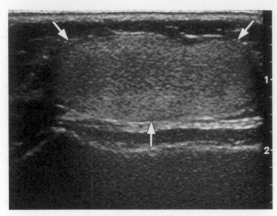

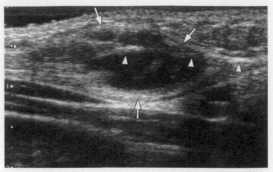

Fig. 16. Lipoblastoma in a 5-month-old girl, who presented with a mobile, rubbery mass in the right upper back, noticed shortly after birth and growing rapidly over previous 3 months. Longitudinal US image of the right scapular region shows a well-defined, homogeneous, hyperechoic mass (*arrows*) confined to the subcutaneous tissues. The increased echogenicity of the mass suggests the presence of fatty tissue. The diagnosis was confirmed on histology.

Fig. 17. Malignant peripheral nerve sheath tumor in an 8-year-old boy with neurofibromatosis type 1 who presented with a 2-month history of nontender, enlarging neck mass. Longitudinal US image of the right side of the anterior neck shows a fusiform, hypoechoic mass (*arrows*) with posterior acoustic enhancement. A hyperechoic cordlike structure, representing a peripheral nerve, is seen entering, coursing through, and exiting the lesion (*arrowheads*), a characteristic feature of peripheral nerve sheath tumors. The diagnosis was confirmed on histology.

neurilemoma) and neurofibroma, and the malignant peripheral nerve sheath tumor.

Schwannoma is usually a solitary, slow-growing tumor of small size (<5 cm) that may present as a soft tissue mass, particularly in the flexor surfaces of the extremities. Because of their eccentric location in relation to the nerve, they are amenable to surgical excision, sparing the normal nerve. Neurofibroma, on the other hand, is inseparable from the normal nerve and therefore its surgical excision includes the adjacent nerve.[41] The localized and diffuse types of neurofibroma are usually solitary lesions not associated with neurofibromatosis type 1. The presence of a plexiform neurofibroma is pathognomonic for neurofibromatosis type 1.

Peripheral nerve sheath tumors may have a characteristic appearance on US, which is of a well-defined hypoechoic fusiform mass with posterior acoustic enhancement, located in an appropriate nerve distribution (**Fig. 17**). A more specific diagnosis can be made when the entering and exiting nerves are identified or rarely in the presence of a complete or incomplete hyperechoic ring within the lesion.[42] Prominent vascularity on color Doppler interrogation has been described with schwannoma and neurofibroma.[42]

Pilomatricoma

Also known as calcifying epithelioma of Malherbe, pilomatricoma is a benign subcutaneous tumor, among the most commonly excised in children. It

arises from hair follicle matrix cells and presents clinically as a slowly growing, superficial hard mass that may be accompanied by bluish discoloration and occasionally ulceration of the overlying skin. It is often of small size, 1.2 cm on average.[43] It is more frequently found in the head and neck but may also present in the trunk and upper extremities.[43]

On US, pilomatricoma is often hyperechoic compared with subcutaneous fat, of heterogeneous texture containing scattered hyperechoic punctate foci, with posterior shadowing caused by calcifications, and a hypoechoic rim (**Fig. 18**).[44] These tumors usually show little vascularity, mainly peripheral, although occasionally central vessels or prominent peripheral vessels can be found with Doppler US. Internal cystic changes and perilesional hyperechogenicity reflecting perilesional inflammatory changes have also been described.

In most instances, the presence of a characteristic US appearance in conjunction with typical clinical findings allows the radiologist to make the diagnosis of pilomatricoma with confidence.

Pseudotumors

This category includes nonneoplastic tumors such as periarticular cysts (ganglion, synovial cyst, and meniscal cyst), hematoma, fat necrosis, and inflammatory masses (cellulitis and abscess – already discussed – and subcutaneous granuloma annulare). US may also be useful in the evaluation of masses in which their origin in the soft tissues or

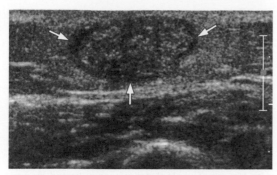

Fig. 18. Pilomatricoma in a 9-year-old girl who presented with a firm, nontender, superficial nodule in the left upper arm, adherent to the dermis. The nodule had been present for about 9 months and had shown gradual growth for the previous 6 months accompanied by blue-purplish discoloration of the overlying skin. Transverse US image of the left upper arm shows a well-defined subcutaneous and cutaneous nodule (*arrows*) of heterogeneous echogenicity with multiple punctate hyperechoic foci and a thin hypoechoic rim. There is subtle increased echogenicity of the adjacent subcutaneous tissues, reflecting a mild reactive inflammatory component. The diagnosis was confirmed on histology.

adjacent bone or cartilaginous structures may not be clear clinically. A common example is in children with asymmetry of the chest wall in whom a prominent costal cartilage may be mistaken for a tumor. In some instances, tumors that are truly originating in the bone may be confused clinically with soft tissue masses, and in the authors' experience this is not rare with osteochondromas, in which US can clearly demonstrate the osseous origin and show the cartilaginous cap characteristic of these exostoses (**Fig. 19**).

Ganglion is a cyst lined by a fibrous capsule lacking synovial cells that contains gelatinous material and often found near but not necessarily communicating with a joint or tendon sheath. In children, ganglia often resolve spontaneously. On US, a ganglion may appear as a simple cyst but it is not uncommon to have internal echoes or septa; it may have a lobulated shape (**Fig. 20**).

Synovial cysts are lined by synovial cells and may represent herniation of synovial membrane through the joint capsule or a bursa distended with fluid; they may communicate with the joint space. The popliteal or Baker cyst is the most common synovial cyst in children and represents an enlargement of the gastrocnemius-semimembranosus bursa, usually of little clinical significance. In contrast to adults and with the exception of those cases seen in patients with JIA, popliteal cysts in children are generally not associated with knee joint effusion or internal knee derangements and often undergo spontaneous involution.[45] On US, popliteal cysts contain anechoic fluid and have smooth margins if they are not related to primary inflammatory pathology, whereas they have a more complex appearance with intraluminal echoes and irregular wall

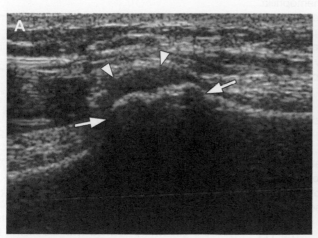
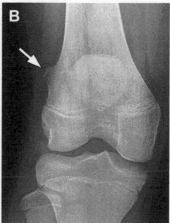

Fig. 19. (*A*) Osteochondroma in a 15-year-old boy with sickle cell disease who presented with a 5-day history of right knee pain attributed to sickle cell crisis. A small, firm, nontender nodule was palpated in the lateral aspect of the right distal thigh on physical examination. Longitudinal US image of the right distal femur shows a bone excrescence (*arrows*) that protrudes into the overlying soft tissues compatible with an osteochondroma. The hypoechoic area seen superficial to the exostosis corresponds to the cartilaginous cap (*arrowheads*). (*B*) Frontal radiograph of the right knee shows characteristic appearance of osteochondroma in the lateral aspect of the distal femur (*arrow*) in correspondence with US findings shown on (*A*). The femoral osteochondroma was believed to be an incidental finding not related to the patient's symptoms.

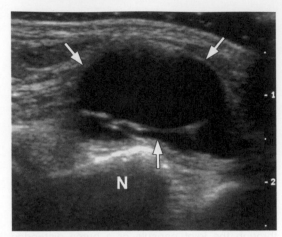

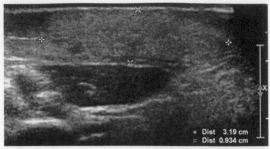

Fig. 20. Ganglion cyst in a 12-year-old girl who presented with a nontender, mobile lump in the dorsum of the left foot. Longitudinal US image of the left shows a well-defined, multiseptated cystic mass (arrows), superficial to the navicular bone (N).

Fig. 21. Subcutaneous fat necrosis in a 3-week-old girl with history of vaginal delivery complicated by perinatal depression, shoulder dystocia necessitating vacuum assistance, and left brachial plexus injury who presented with 2 hard lumps in the right shoulder and axillary regions. Longitudinal US image of the right shoulder region shows a well-defined hyperechoic, homogeneous mass in the subcutaneous tissues (between cursors). The nodules gradually decreased in size and resolved spontaneously in a few weeks.

thickening if they are associated with inflammatory arthropathies or internal knee derangement.

Meniscal cyst is a parameniscal or intrameniscal collection of fluid in association with a meniscal tear. On US, meniscal cysts may appear as simple cysts but may also have a more complex appearance because of internal septa or mixed echogenicity.

Hematomas are often diagnosed clinically but imaging may be indicated in symptomatic cases, in children without a clear history of trauma or in those with bleeding disorders such as hemophilia. The US appearance of hematomas varies depending on age of the blood. Hematomas appear as hyperechoic masses in the acute phase, show progressive decrease in echogenicity in a few hours, and become anechoic in a few days.

Fat necrosis is a self-limited entity that often presents clinically as a small, firm, nontender subcutaneous nodule. Causes for fat necrosis include trauma, cold exposure, iatrogenic injections, autoimmune disorders, vasculitis, and sickle cell disease. A common age of presentation in children is the first weeks of life, and hypoxia, hypothermia, and obstetric injury seem to play a main role. Frequent locations include the soft tissues overlying bone prominences in the shoulders, back, buttocks, thighs, and cheeks.[46] The US appearance is variable although typically fat necrosis appears as a hyperechoic subcutaneous nodule with fuzzy margins and little vascularity, mainly peripheral (Fig. 21).

Subcutaneous granuloma annulare is a self-limited, rapidly growing, nontender, inflammatory dermatosis of unknown cause with characteristic

formation of so-called pallisading granulomas on pathology.[47] It is more commonly seen in children between the ages of 2 and 5 years and usual locations include the extremities, especially the pretibial subcutaneous tissues, and the scalp in the region of the occiput. On US, subcutaneous granuloma annulare appears as an ill-defined hypoechoic solid mass,[48] with variable vascularity (Fig. 22). Biopsy is often required for final diagnosis.

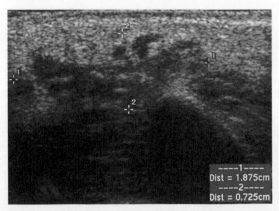

Fig. 22. Subcutaneous granuloma annulare in a 4-year-old girl who presented with a 3-month history of firm, nonmobile, nontender mass in the right forearm. Although the mass showed initial growth, it seemed to have been decreasing in size over the previous 2 weeks. Transverse US image of the right forearm shows an irregular hypoechoic mass (between cursors) in the subcutaneous tissues abutting the underlying fascial planes. The diagnosis was confirmed on histology.

SUMMARY

US plays a major role in the evaluation of musculoskeletal pathology in the pediatric age group because of its multiple advantages; it should be used in a rational fashion along with other imaging modalities, particularly MR imaging. US is frequently the only imaging modality required for diagnosis and monitoring of musculoskeletal pathology. In those instances in which US is not diagnostic, it is often useful for planning further imaging or for guidance of interventional procedures.

REFERENCES

1. Bellah R. Ultrasound in pediatric musculoskeletal disease: techniques and applications. Radiol Clin North Am 2001;39(4):597–618.

2. Jacobson JA. Musculoskeletal sonography and MR imaging. A role for both imaging methods. Radiol Clin North Am 1999;37(4):713–35.

3. Jemec GB, Gniadecka M, Ulrich J. Ultrasound in dermatology. Part I. High frequency ultrasound. Eur J Dermatol 2000;10(6):492–7.

4. Walker FO, Cartwright MS, Wiesler ER, et al. Ultrasound of nerve and muscle. Clin Neurophysiol 2004;115(3):495–507.

5. Lee JC, Healy JC. Normal sonographic anatomy of the wrist and hand. Radiographics 2005;25(6): 1577–90.

6. Grassi W, Filippucci E, Busilacchi P. Musculoskeletal ultrasound. Best Pract Res Clin Rheumatol 2004; 18(6):813–26.

7. Connolly DJ, Berman L, McNally EG. The use of beam angulation to overcome anisotropy when viewing human tendon with high frequency linear array ultrasound. Br J Radiol 2001;74(878):183–5.

8. Silvestri E, Martinoli C, Derchi L, et al. Echotexture of peripheral nerves: correlation between US and histological findings and criteria to differentiate tendons. Radiology 1995;197(1):291–6.

9. Chau CLF, Griffith JF. Musculoskeletal infections: ultrasound appearances. Clin Radiol 2005;60(2): 149–59.

10. Robben SGF. Ultrasonography of musculoskeletal infections in children. Eur Radiol 2004;14(Suppl 4): L65–77.

11. Horton LK, Jacobson JA, Powell A, et al. Sonography and radiography of soft-tissue foreign bodies. AJR Am J Roentgenol 2001;176(5):1155–9.

12. Kothari NA, Pelchovitz DJ, Meyer JS. Imaging of musculoskeletal infections. Radiol Clin North Am 2001;39(4):653–71.

13. Zamzam MM. The role of ultrasound in differentiating septic arthritis from transient synovitis of the hip in children. J Pediatr Orthop B 2006;15(6):418–22.

14. Mathews CJ, Coakley G. Septic arthritis: current diagnostic and therapeutic algorithm. Curr Opin Rheumatol 2008;20(4):457–62.

15. Offiah AC. Acute osteomyelitis, septic arthritis and discitis: differences between neonates and older children. Eur J Radiol 2006;60(2):221–32.

16. Zawin JK, Hoffer FA, Rand FF, et al. Joint effusion in children with an irritable hip: US diagnosis and aspiration. Radiology 1993;187(2):459–63.

17. Weiss JE, Ilowite NT. Juvenile idiopathic arthritis. Pediatr Clin North Am 2005;52(2):413–42.

18. Manners PJ, Bower C. Worldwide prevalence of juvenile arthritis: why does it vary so much? J Rheumatol 2002;29(7):1520–30.

19. Hashkes PJ, Laxer RM. Medical treatment of juvenile idiopathic arthritis. JAMA 2005;294(13):1671–84.

20. Borchers AT, Selmi C, Cheema G, et al. Juvenile idiopathic arthritis. Autoimmun Rev 2006;5(4): 279–98.

21. Selvaag A, Flato B, Dale K, et al. Radiographic and clinical outcome in early juvenile rheumatoid arthritis and juvenile spondiloarthropathy: a 3-year prospective study. J Rheumatol 2006;33(7):1382–91.

22. Johnson K. Imaging of juvenile idiopathic arthritis. Pediatr Radiol 2006;36(8):743–58.

23. Rooney M, McAllister C, Burns J. Ankle disease in juvenile idiopathic arthritis: ultrasound findings in clinically swollen ankles. J Rheumatol 2009;36(8):1725–9.

24. Acharya S. Hemophilic joint disease–current perspective and potential future strategies. Transfus Apher Sci 2008;38(1):49–55.

25. Klukowska A, Czyrny Z, Laguna P, et al. Correlation between clinical, radiological and ultrasonographical image of knee joints in children with haemophilia. Haemophilia 2001;7(3):286–92.

26. Brisse H, Orbach D, Klijanienko J, et al. Imaging and diagnostic strategy of soft tissue tumors in children. Eur Radiol 2006;16(5):1147–64.

27. Fletcher CDM, Unni KK, Martins F, editors. World Health Organization classification of tumours. Pathology and genetics of tumours of soft tissue and bone. Lyon, France: IARC Press; 2002.

28. Nikolaidis P, Gabriel HA, Lamba AR, et al. Sonographic appearance of nodular fasciitis. J Ultrasound Med 2006;25(2):281–5.

29. Bedi DG, John SD, Swischuk LE. Fibromatosis colli of infancy: variability of sonographic appearance. J Clin Ultrasound 1998;26(7):345–8.

30. Deeg KH, Güttler N, Windschall D. Diagnosis of fibromatosis colli via color-coded duplex sonography in 13 infants. Ultraschall Med 2008;29(Suppl 5):226–32.

31. Wiswell TE, Davis J, Cunningham BE, et al. Infantile myofibromatosis: the most common fibrous tumor of infancy. J Pediatr Surg 1988;23(4):315–8.

32. Soper JR, De Silva M. Infantile myofibromatosis: a radiologic review. Pediatr Radiol 1993;23(3): 189–94.

33. Koujok K, Ruiz RE, Hernandez RJ. Myofibromatosis: imaging characteristics. Pediatr Radiol 2005;35(4): 374–80.

34. Lee JC, Thomas JM, Phillips S, et al. Aggressive fibromatosis: MRI features with pathologic correlation. AJR Am J Roentgenol 2006;186(1):247–54.

35. Spiegel DA, Dormans JP, Meyer JS, et al. Aggressive fibromatosis from infancy to adolescence. J Pediatr Orthop 1999;19(6):776–84.

36. Bernathova M, Felfernig M, Rachbauer F, et al. Sonographic imaging of abdominal and extraabdominal desmoids. Ultraschall Med 2008;29(5):515–9.

37. Miller GG, Yanchar NL, Magee JF, et al. Lipoblastoma and liposarcoma in children: an analysis of 9 cases and a review of the literature. Can J Surg 1998;41(6):455–8.

38. Inampudi P, Jacobson JA, Fessell DP, et al. Soft-tissue lipomas: accuracy of sonography in diagnosis with pathologic correlation. Radiology 2004;233(3): 763–7.

39. Ahuja AT, King AD, Kew J, et al. Head and neck lipomas: sonographic appearance. AJNR Am J Neuroradiol 1998;19(3):505–8.

40. Moholkar S, Sebire NJ, Roebuck DJ. Radiological-pathological correlation in lipoblastoma and lipoblastomatosis. Pediatr Radiol 2006;36(8):851–6.

41. Murphey MD, Smith WS, Smith SE, et al. From the archives of the AFIP. Imaging of musculoskeletal neurogenic tumors: radiologic-pathologic correlation. Radiographics 1999;19(5):1253–80.

42. Beggs I. Sonographic appearances of nerve tumors. J Clin Ultrasound 1999;27(7):363–8.

43. Pirouzmanesh A, Reinisch JF, Gonzalez-Gomez I, et al. Pilomatrixoma: a review of 346 cases. Plast Reconstr Surg 2003;112(7):1784–9.

44. Lim HW, Im SA, Lim GY, et al. Pilomatricomas in children: imaging characteristics with pathologic correlation. Pediatr Radiol 2007;37(6):549–55.

45. De Maeseneer M, Debaere C, Desprechins B, et al. Popliteal cysts in children: prevalence, appearance and associated findings at MR imaging. Pediatr Radiol 1999;29(8):605–9.

46. Tsai TS, Evans HA, Donnelly LF, et al. Fat necrosis after trauma: a benign cause of palpable lumps in children. AJR Am J Roentgenol 1997;169(6):1623–6.

47. McDermott MB, Lind AC, Marley EF, et al. Deep granuloma annulare (pseudorheumatoid nodule) in children: clinicopathologic study of 35 cases. Pediatr Dev Pathol 1998;1(4):300–8.

48. Abiezzi SS, Miller LS. The use of ultrasound for the diagnosis of soft-tissue masses in children. J Pediatr Orthop 1995;15(5):566–73.

Vascular Anomalies

Josée Dubois, MSc, MD, FRCP(C)[a,b,]*, Françoise Rypens, MD[a,b]

KEYWORDS
- Vascular anomalies • Ultrasound • Hemangiomas
- Vascular malformation

Since 1980, many articles have tried to clarify the confusion that has prevailed in vascular anomalies. Despite these attempts, improper terminology is still often used, leading to inappropriate descriptions of imaging studies and sometimes to misdiagnosis and mismanagement of vascular anomalies.[1]

A biologic classification has helped to resolve the nosology of vascular anomalies in approximately 90% of lesions. This classification was first described by Mulliken in Glowacki in 1982, and subsequently modified and adopted by the International Society for the Study of Vascular Anomalies (ISSVA) in Rome in 1996.[2,3]

Vascular anomalies are classified into 2 distinct biologic groups: the vascular tumors, characterized by initial cellular proliferation and hyperplasia; and the vascular malformations, featuring dysmorphogenesis and normal endothelial turnover.

All physicians, particularly dermatologists, pathologists, radiologists, plastic surgeons, and orthopedists, are strongly encouraged to adopt this classification and stop using the confusing old descriptors. Proper terminology is essential for an interdisciplinary approach to establishing a precise diagnosis, for planning adequate management, and for collecting relevant data.

Most vascular anomalies have a typical clinical appearance and can be diagnosed without imaging. However, when lesions have an atypical appearance or evolution, are located deeply or adjacent to a vital structure, or are associated with a coagulopathy or a functional disorder and require treatment, imaging is needed.

The initial primary imaging modality is Doppler ultrasound (US). It is widely available and remains the best modality to assess the hemodynamics of the vascular lesion and distinguish low- and fast-flow malformations. Magnetic resonance imaging (MRI) is the best technique for evaluating the extent of the lesions and their relationship to adjacent structures.

This article reviews the clinical and the Doppler US features of soft-tissue vascular anomalies, including a brief summary of the available therapeutic options and their relative indications.

CLASSIFICATION OF VASCULAR ANOMALIES

Classification of vascular anomalies is based on the histologic appearance of the abnormal channel, flow characteristics, and clinical behavior.[2] It was updated during the 1996 meeting of the ISSVA (**Table 1**). Vascular tumors are characterized by initial cellular proliferation and hyperplasia. Infantile hemangioma is the most frequent vascular tumor in infancy. Other vascular tumors reported in children include congenital hemangioma (ie, noninvoluting congenital

[a] Department of Radiology, Radio-Oncology and Nuclear Medicine, University of Montreal, 2900 Edouard-Montpetit Boulevard, Montreal, Quebec H3T 1J4, Canada
[b] Department of Medical Imaging, CHU Sainte-Justine Mother and Child University Hospital Center, 3175 Cote Ste-Catherine Road, Montreal, Quebec H3T 1C5, Canada
* Corresponding author. Department of Medical Imaging, CHU Sainte-Justine, 3175 Cote Ste-Catherine Road, Montreal, Quebec H3T 1C5, Canada.
E-mail address: josee-dubois@ssss.gouv.qc.ca (J. Dubois).

Ultrasound Clin 4 (2009) 471–495
doi:10.1016/j.cult.2009.11.002

Table 1
Vascular anomalies

Tumors	Vascular Malformations	
Hemangiomas	Simple Malformations	Combined Malformations
Others	Capillary	AVFs
	Lymphatic	AVM
	Venous	Capillary venous malformation
	Arterial	Capillary lymphaticovenous malformation
		Lymphaticovenous malformation
		Capillary AVM
		Capillary lymphaticoarteriovenous malformation

hemangioma [NICH] or rapidly involuting congenital hemangioma [RICH]), hemangioendothelioma, tufted angioma, pyogenic granuloma, or sarcoma.

Vascular malformations are localized or diffuse errors of embryonic development at some stage of either vasculogenesis or angiogenesis. They are presumably present at birth but most of them become evident only during the teen years and persist throughout life. They are the most often encountered vascular anomalies.

Vascular malformations are classified as slow-flow malformations, including capillary malformations, venous malformations, lymphatic malformations, capillary venous malformations (CVM), and capillary lymphatic venous malformations, and as high-flow malformations, including

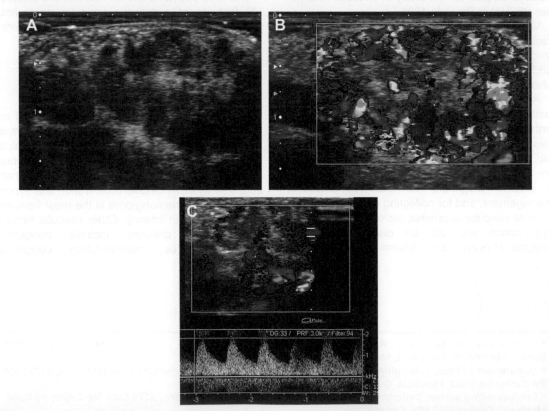

Fig. 1. A 1-month-old baby with cheek lesion and normal overlying skin. (*A*) US reveals a hypoechoic polylobulated lesion. (*B*) Color Doppler shows hypervascularity. (*C*) High systolic peak greater than 2 kHz with low RI is shown. Diagnosis: infantile hemangioma.

arteriovenous fistula (AVF) and arteriove-nous malformations (AVM). Complex combined malformations are found in several syndromes: Klippel-Trénaunay, Parkes Weber, blue rubber bleb nevus, Proteus, and Maffucci.

DOPPLER US TECHNIQUES

US examination includes an initial B-mode evaluation followed by color Doppler and spectral analysis with duplex Doppler. It should be performed using an appropriate and reproducible technique by an experienced radiologist with knowledge of the clinical history and symptoms. A high-frequency linear array transducer (5–12 MHz) is optimal, depending on the depth of the lesion.

On B-mode evaluation the radiologist should characterize the borders of the lesion (well-defined or not), and assess the presence or absence of solid tissues, the echogenicity of the lesion relative to the adjacent normal soft tissues or muscle (hypoechoic, hyperechoic, or heterogeneous). The presence of calcification, cystic components, and visible vessels in or around the lesion must be noted. The compressibility or the expansion of the lesion during a Valsalva maneuver should be assessed during the examination.

Color Doppler US is performed using a soft-tissue preset with a low-pulse frequency and a wall filter. Pulse-repetition frequency is increased only if aliasing is observed. Color Doppler US is helpful to quantify the vessel density by counting the number of color Doppler dots within an area of 1 cm^2. This quantification is done in the portion

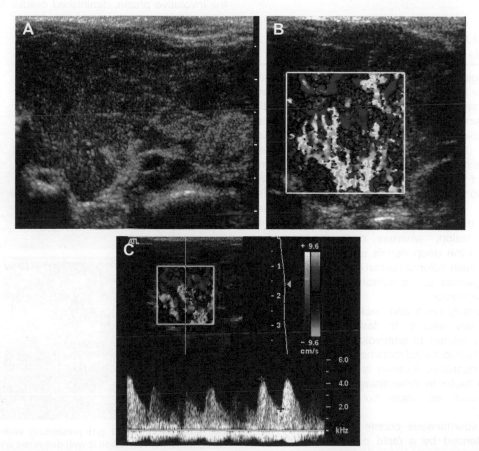

Fig. 2. A 9-month-old boy with an enlarging preauricular mass. (*A*) US shows a hypoechoic mass. (*B*) Color Doppler shows hypervascularity. (*C*) High-velocity arteries with low resistance typical of hemangioma. Diagnosis: infantile hemangioma.

of the lesion with the greatest vascularity. By using this approach, the vascularization can be classified as follows: low vascularization = fewer than 2 vessels per square centimeter; moderate vascularization = 2 to 4 vessels per square centimeter; high vascularization = 5 or more vessels per square centimeter.[4]

Pulsed Doppler sonography is also performed, with maximal systolic Doppler shift being measured in kilohertz because angle correction cannot be accurate for most examinations. It is instrumental to assess the arterial and venous flow and the presence of AVFs. Measurement of arterial resistive index (RI) is helpful to document objectively the arterial resistance. RI is defined as peak systolic Doppler shift/end-diastolic Doppler shift/peak systolic Doppler shift.

The presence of a feeding artery with an increased diastolic flow associated with enlarged veins caused by an increased venous return and pulsatile venous flow is typically observed in AVFs.

VASCULAR TUMORS
Infantile Hemangiomas

Hemangiomas of infancy are the most common vascular tumor of infancy. The incidence of infantile hemangiomas is estimated to be 10% to 12% in full-term babies, and more than 20% in premature babies, especially those weighing less than 1.5 kg. There is a 3:1 female predominance.[5] Infantile hemangiomas usually appear in the first week of life and are located in the head and neck (60%), the trunk (25%), and the extremities (15%). Clinically, superficial hemangiomas involve the superficial dermis with a red "strawberry" lesion, whereas deep hemangiomas involving the deep dermis and subcutis present with a bluish color or normal overlying skin. Mixed hemangiomas are a combination of superficial and deep lesions.

Regarding head and neck hemangiomas, the distribution seems to favor particular sites, possibly related to embryologic fusion lines and facial developmental metameres.[2] The importance of the anatomic location is well recognized as a major factor in determining potential complications, such as visual compromise in orbital lesions.[6–8]

The spontaneous course of hemangiomas is characterized by a rapid postnatal proliferation of 3 to 12 months' duration, a variable length stability plateau, followed by a slow involution (2–10 years).

Multiple cutaneous hemangiomas (>5) are associated with concomitant visceral lesions. The most common visceral lesion is the infantile hepatic hemangioma. Hepatic hemangiomas may be asymptomatic or may result in congestive heart failure related to the arteriovenous shunt.

Abnormalities associated with infantile hemangiomas include central nervous system anomalies (Dandy-Walker, microcephaly, agenesis of the corpus callosum, filum terminale syndrome), ocular anomalies (microphthalmos, cataract, optic nerve hypoplasia), congenital cardiovascular malformations (aortic coarctation), visceral malformations (biliary atresia, imperforated anus, bladder extrophy), limb hypertrophy, and cleft palate. The PHACE association consists of posterior fossa brain malformations, hemangiomas, arterial and cardiac anomalies, coarctation of the aorta, and eye anomalies.[9]

Histologically, during the proliferative phase a hemangioma consists of plump, hyperplastic endothelial cells, pericytes, and dendritic cells, and contains a large number of mast cells. During the involutive phase, diminished cellular turnover

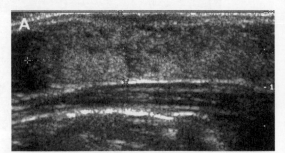
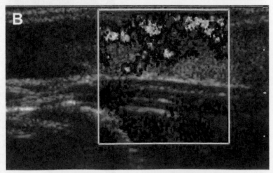

Fig. 3. A 4-month-old girl presenting with a soft-tissue mass. (*A*) The lesion is well delimited and hyperechoic compared with the adjacent subcutaneous fat. (*B*) Color Doppler reveals a hypervascular lesion. Diagnosis: infantile hemangioma.

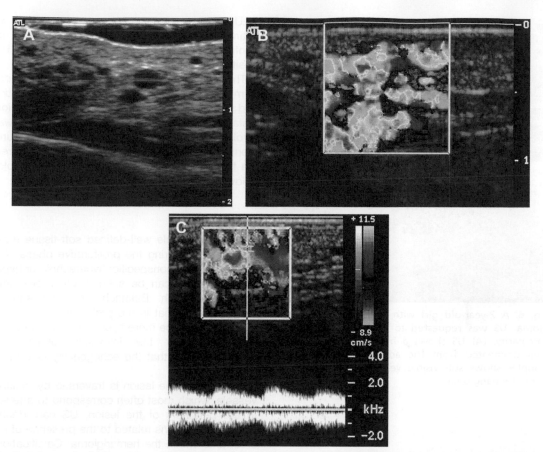

Fig. 4. A 3-month-old boy presenting with a growing palpable pulsatile mass, present since birth. (*A*) US shows a hyperechoic subcutaneous mass with compressible vessels (only a part of the mass is shown). (*B*) Color Doppler shows a hypervascular lesion. (*C*) Pulsed Doppler shows high-velocity arteries with low resistance. Diagnosis: hemangioma.

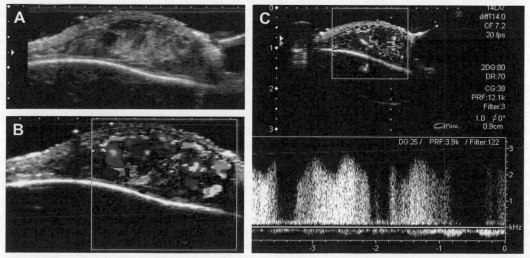

Fig. 5. An 8-month-old girl presenting with a soft occipital mass. (*A*) US shows a heterogeneous well-delimitated subcutaneous mass distinct from the adjacent skull bone. (*B*) Color Doppler shows a hypervascular lesion. (*C*) Waveform shows arteries with high velocity and low resistance compatible with microfistulae. Diagnosis: infantile hemangioma.

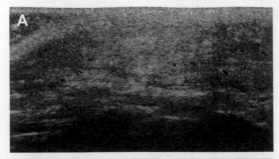

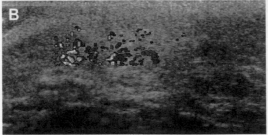

Fig. 6. A 2-year-old girl with an ulcerated hemangioma. US was requested to evaluate the residual vascularity. (A) US shows a hyperechoic lesion not well delineated from the adjacent fat. (B) Color Doppler shows still visible vessels. Diagnosis: involuting hemangioma.

and progressive deposition of perivascular and interlobular fibrous tissue are observed. Recent studies of the pathogenesis of vascular diseases focus on the role of cell proliferation as a determinant of vessel cellularity. There is evidence to suggest that vascular structure and lesion formation are determined by a balance between cell death by apoptosis and cell proliferation. During the involutive phase of hemangiomas, apoptosis of endothelial cells announces the switch from uncontrolled growth to spontaneous tumor resorption.[10]

Recent advances in the physiology of angiogenesis have shown the role of basic fibroblast growth factor (BFGF), proliferating cell nuclear antigen, type IV collagenase, E-selectin, and monocytic chemoattractant protein during the proliferating phase. Conversely, during the involutive phase, there is an increase of the tissue inhibitor metalloproteinase (inhibiting new blood vessel formation). Accordingly, BFGF is increased in the urine initially and tends to decrease as the hemangioma begins to regress. These markers monitor the activity of angiogenesis within the hemangioma. Research is active in histopathology and molecular phenotyping.[10,11] North and colleagues[12] have identified

GLU1 as an immunohistochemical marker for infantile hemangiomas. The diagnosis can be confirmed when the immunophenotype GLU1 is positive.

The most important predictors of poor short-term outcomes, as measured by complication and treatment rates, are large size of the lesion, facial location, or segmental morphology. Airway involvement, ulceration, or permanent disfigurement may then occur.[1,3,4] If treatment is required, the first line is based on steroids or propranolol, followed by interferon, vincristine, or surgery.

US imaging

On US, a variable well-defined soft-tissue mass can be seen during the proliferative phase. The echogenicity is nonspecific; hyperechoic or hypoechoic lesions can be seen in the proliferative phase. Although Bakhach and colleagues[13] have reported that in the proliferative phase the lesion tends to be more hypoechoic and become hyperechoic in the involutive phase, the authors believe that the echogenicity is variable (Figs. 1–3).

Sometimes, the lesion is traversed by multiple vessels, which most often correspond to arteries. In the periphery of the lesion, US can identify some dilated veins related to the presence of microshunts within the hemangioma. Calcifications are never observed in soft-tissue infantile hemangioma.

Color Doppler US is important for making the diagnosis of hemangioma and recognizing mimicking conditions. The lesion displays an increased color flow caused by numerous arteries and veins. The high vessel density (>5 vessels/cm^2) with high Doppler shift (>2 kHz) and low resistance are characteristic of infantile hemangiomas (Fig. 4).[6] Paltiel and colleagues[14] have reported high vessel density in 41 patients out of 49, with mean peak arterial flow velocity and an RI estimated at 28.4 ± 5.0 cm/s and 0.54 ± 0.02, respectively. Arteriovenous shunting can be seen on spectral Doppler analysis and is frequently misinterpreted as indicating an AVM (Fig. 5).

During the involutive phase, infantile hemangioma appears as a sonographically heterogeneous mass that becomes hyperechoic. The mass decreases in volume with a reduced number of vessel density. Sometimes a hypoechoic residual lesion with a high Doppler shift in the remaining vessels can be seen but an increase of the RI is observed (mean: 0.7) (Fig. 6).[13]

In conclusion, the presence of a distinct mass at sonography, the high vessel density, and the low RI with Doppler are the most important diagnostic

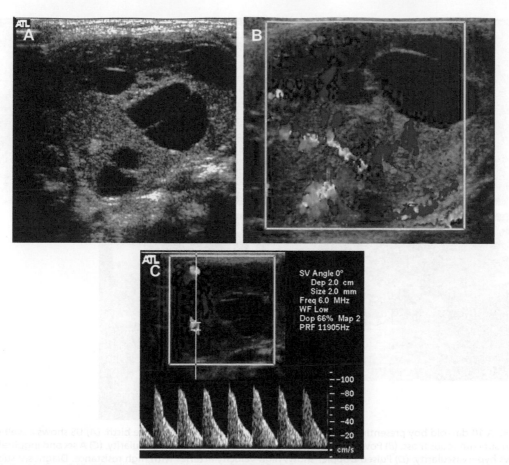

Fig. 7. An 11-day-old baby girl presenting with a left cervical mass. (*A*) US shows a heterogeneous mass containing cysts with slightly hyperechoic areas. (*B*) Color Doppler shows the solid part contains numerous vessels. (*C*) Tumoral vessels show high-velocity systolic peak and high resistance. Diagnosis: fibrosarcoma.

criteria of infantile hemangioma; these criteria can also be used to monitor lesion evolution.

Differential diagnosis

Some vascular tumors can mimic infantile hemangiomas. When the clinical features and the imaging criteria are not correlated, a biopsy has to be performed to exclude infantile myofibromatosis, fibrosarcoma (**Fig. 7**), rhabdomyosarcoma, metastatic neuroblastoma (**Fig. 8**), pyogenic granuloma (**Fig. 10**), or other tumors (**Figs. 9, 10**). These tumors rarely have the high vessel density and high Doppler shift with low RI, except the pyogenic granuloma (**Fig. 11**). Pyogenic granuloma is commonly confused with infantile hemangioma, but is rarely seen before 6 months of age.

Congenital Hemangiomas

First introduced by Boon and colleagues[15] in 1996, congenital hemangiomas are divided into 2 types: the noninvoluting hemangioma (NICH), which grows proportionally with the child without involution, and the rapidly involuting hemangioma (RICH), which regresses completely within 14 months after birth. These congenital hemangiomas are GLU1 negative.[16,17] They are fully grown at birth with an equal sex distribution, are usually solitary, and have a similar average diameter and a predilection for the same cutaneous locations as infantile hemangiomas (head or limbs near a joint). NICH has a typical appearance: the color is violaceous with multiple tiny or coarse telangiectasias, often with a surrounding pale halo, and sometimes a central ulceration, linear scar, or central nodule.[18] The treatment of RICH is conservative considering its rapid involution. Regarding

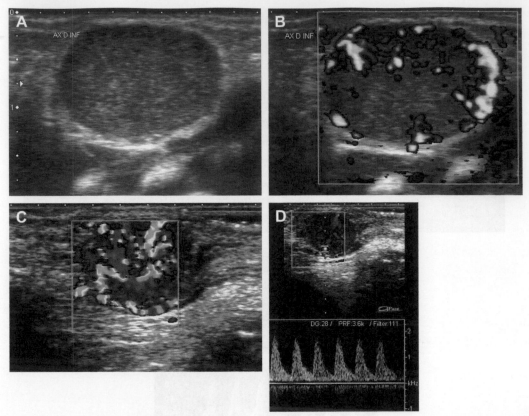

Fig. 8. A 10-day-old boy presenting with an axillary mass increasing in size since birth. (*A*) US shows a well-delineated subcutaneous mass. (*B*) Power Doppler shows a mass with peripheral vascularity. (*C*) A second inguinal mass shows hypervascularity. (*D*) Pulsed Doppler shows high-velocity arteries with high resistance. Diagnosis: subcutaneous metastasis of neuroblastoma.

NICH, surgical removal is the treatment of choice, when necessary.

US imaging
NICH NICH can display the same appearance as infantile hemangioma, with high systolic flow, low RI, and a high vessel density,[19] but several differences can be observed at US. The lesion is more commonly heterogeneous than infantile hemangioma because of the presence of calcifications or intravascular thrombi. Most of the visible vessels are made of venous ectasia. Microarteriovenous shunting is frequently identified, and sometimes arterial aneurysms are present (**Figs. 12–14**).

RICH RICH is hypoechoic, heterogeneous, and mainly confined to the subcutaneous fat.[20] Multiple vessels with arterial and venous flow can be seen through the lesion. Most of them have the same characteristics of high vessel density

and high Doppler shift as infantile hemangiomas.[19] Microarteriovenous shunt can be seen. Contrary to the infantile hemangioma, calcification can be identified (**Figs. 15, 16**).

Hemangioendothelioma

Kaposiform hemangioendothelioma is a rare tumor. It may be congenital or develop during infancy. Later presentations are reported in the literature.[21] This tumor is a tender, red, ill-defined mass generally located on the trunk, limbs, and retroperitoneum. Kaposiform hemangioendotheliomas are aggressive, composed of irregular lobules, with a lacy network of sheet cells infiltrating the dermis and the subcutaneous fat. The tumor cells are spindle-shaped endothelial cells, with diminished pericytes and mast cells, microthrombi, and hemosiderin deposits. Dilated, hyperplastic, lymphaticoid channels are predominant in the tumor. The immunohistochemical

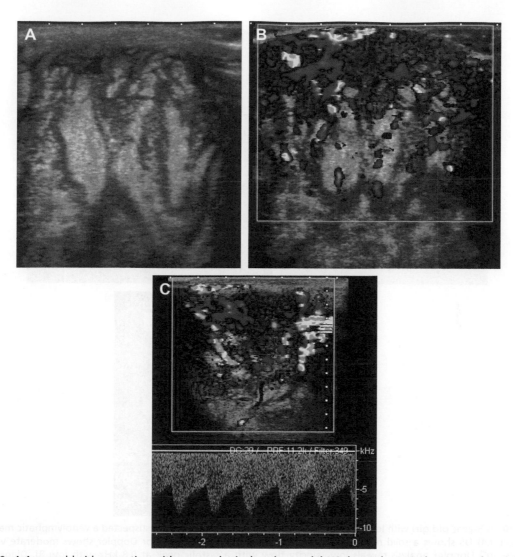

Fig. 9. A 4-year-old girl presenting with an exophytic dorsal mass. (*A*) US shows the typical pattern of a schwannoma with hyper- and hypoechoic linear structures. (*B*) Color Doppler illustrates the hypervascularity of the tumor. (*C*) Arteries are numerous with high systolic peak and low resistance. Diagnosis: schwannoma.

marker GLU1 is negative. These hemangioendotheliomas either spontaneously shrink and disappear or persist with progressive worsening.

Hemangioendotheliomas can be associated with the Kasabach-Merritt phenomenon (KMP), consisting of severe thrombocytopenia, microangiopathic hemolytic anemia, and localized consumptive coagulopathy. KMP is a severe condition, with mortality ranging from 20% to 30%. Most patients with KMP do not have classic hemangiomas but either kaposiform hemangioendotheliomas (also called spindle cell

hemangiomas) or tufted angiomas.[22,23] Enjolras and colleagues[24] have reported 41 patients with residual lesions after the resolution of thrombocytopenia and coagulopathy. Because of its mortality, KMP requires aggressive treatment with antiangiogenesis drugs and sometimes embolization also.

US imaging
On US, hemangioendotheliomas appear as ill-defined, infiltrative soft-tissue masses with variable echogenicity. Most of them show evidence

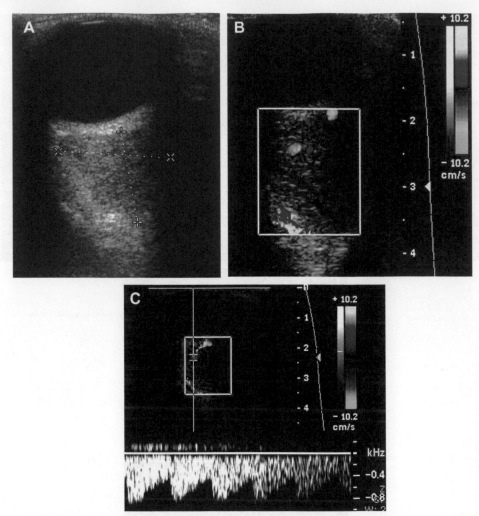

Fig. 10. A 5-year-old girl with left orbital ptosis. Computed tomography scan suspected a venolymphatic malformation. (*A*) US shows a solid mass (*cursors*) posterior to the globe. (*B*) Color Doppler shows moderate vessel density. (*C*) Doppler analysis reveals low-velocity flow with a systolic peak at 0.8 kHz with low RI. Diagnosis: rhabdomyosarcoma.

of necrotic areas with cavities and calcifications within the lesion. Doppler US displays a high, moderate, or low vessel density, and most hemangioendotheliomas have a high Doppler shift of more than 2 kHz with low RI.[25] Arteriovenous shunting is rarely seen (**Figs. 17** and **18**).

Tufted Angioma

Tufted angioma is a rare benign superficial vascular tumor, located in the skin of the neck and trunk. It can be associated with KMP. Most

tufted angiomas require a biopsy to confirm the diagnosis.

US imaging

The lesion is superficial and ill-defined with skin thickening. The lesion appears hyperechoic or hypoechoic on B-mode imaging. The vessel density and systolic Doppler shift (0.7–1 kHz) are typically low.[25] No calcification or shunt is seen within the lesion (**Fig. 19**).

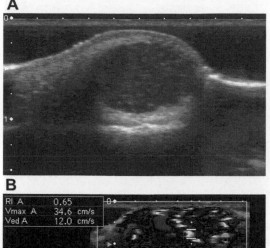

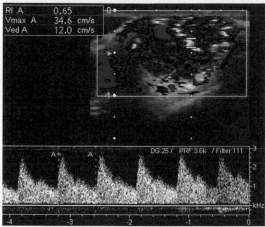

Fig. 11. A 15-year-old boy presenting with a small mass of the left ear lobule. (*A*) US shows a well-delimitated hypoechoic superficial mass located in the subcutaneous tissue. (*B*) Doppler reveals numerous vessels inside the mass with high-velocity and low-resistance arteries. Diagnosis: pyogenic granuloma.

VASCULAR MALFORMATIONS

Low-flow vascular malformations include venous, capillary, lymphatic, and various combined malformations.

Venous Malformations

Venous malformation is the most common vascular anomaly. It is a slow-flow malformation with an abnormal venous network. The confusing term "cavernous hemangioma" is no longer appropriate and should not be used.

Venous malformations are characterized clinically by a soft, compressible, nonpulsatile tissue mass. The overlying skin usually has a bluish tint, but occasionally may appear normal. The main locations of venous malformations are the head and neck (40%), trunk (20%), and extremities (40%), but they can be found anywhere.[3,26,27] Characteristically, venous malformations expand after Valsalva maneuver or if they are in a dependent position, and may be compressed by gentle pressure. They grow proportionally with the patient but can enlarge during puberty and pregnancy from hormonal influence. They do not regress. Although most venous malformations are in the skin and subcutaneous tissues, they also often involve underlying muscles, bones, and abdominal viscera. Most venous malformations are solitary, but multiple cutaneous or visceral lesions can occur. Venous malformations are associated sometimes with bony abnormalities or are part of a syndrome (Klippel-Trénaunay, Gorham, Maffucci, blue rubber bleb nevus syndrome).

Symptoms are related to size and location. Swelling and pain are common in venous malformations, often from phlebothrombosis.[28] Intraoral venous malformations can bleed, distort dentition, cause speech problems, or obstruct the upper airway and pharynx. Blood stagnation within a venous malformation can induce localized intravascular coagulopathy, as shown by positive D-dimer levels and normal or low platelets and fibrinogen values.[29]

The locus for autosomal dominant multiple cutaneous and mucosal venous malformations, VMCM1, was mapped to chromosome 9p21 [30] and involves a mutation in the endothelial cell specific receptor tyrosine kinase TIE-2.[31] This mutation is likely to occur in vascular anomalies. Venous malformations and glomus cells show linkage to chromosome 1p21–p22.[32]

Histopathologic examination of venous malformations shows thin-walled, dilated, spongelike channels varying in size from capillary to cavernous dimensions, with sparse smooth muscle cells, adventitial fibrosis, thrombosis, and phleboliths. Smooth muscle actin staining reveals muscle in clumps instead of the normal smooth muscular architecture. The mural muscular abnormality is probably responsible for the gradual expansion of venous malformations.

Asymptomatic venous malformations should be treated conservatively. Extensive lower and upper extremity venous malformations should be first treated with elastic stockings. When the venous malformation causes aesthetic problems, pain, or functional problems, sclerotherapy is recommended. Surgery is performed after sclerotherapy when the treatment is incomplete or when aesthetic concerns require correction.

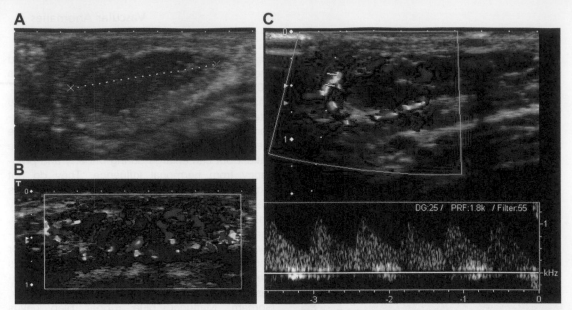

Fig. 12. A 1-year-old girl with a thoracic mass present since 2 months of age. (*A*) US shows a subcutaneous mass with a hypoechoic center and echogenic halo. (*B*) Color Doppler performed at 2 months of age shows diffuse hypervascularity. (*C*) Color Doppler performed at 1 year of age shows persistent peripheral arteries with high velocity and low resistance. Diagnosis: NICH.

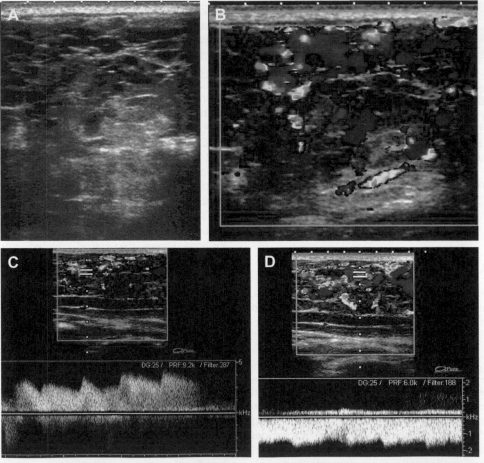

Fig. 13. An 11-year-old girl with a stable cervical lesion present since birth. (*A*) US shows a heterogeneous lesion with vessels inside the thickened subcutaneous tissue. (*B*) Color Doppler shows hypervascularity. (*C*) Pulsed Doppler shows numerous high-velocity low-resistance vessels. (*D*) Abnormal dilated pulsatile veins are easily detected. Diagnosis: NICH.

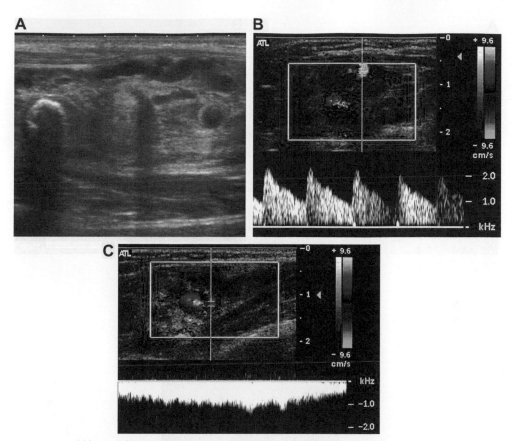

Fig. 14. A 10-year-old boy with a congenital mass of the forearm. (*A*) US shows a heterogeneous echogenic mass containing phleboliths and peripheral serpiginous dilated vessels. (*B*) Color Doppler performed at the age of 3 years shows high-velocity and low-resistance arteries. (*C*) Color Doppler performed at the age of 3 years showed large visible veins. Diagnosis: NICH.

US imaging

The venous malformations can be classified in 2 types: cavitary and dysplastic. The cavitary venous malformation is common. B-mode examination shows a compressible hypoechoic and heterogeneous infiltrative lesion.[14,27] After applying compression, US displays the movement of blood into the cavities. Phleboliths are identified in less than 20% of cases (**Figs. 20** and **21**).[27] Doppler US typically shows monophasic low-velocity flow. Doppler flow may be difficult to obtain because flow is below threshold or because of thrombosis. Dynamic maneuvers, such as Valsalva or manual compression, are sometimes necessary to induce a visible Doppler flow (**Fig. 22**). Arterial flow can be observed in the lesion in capillaries in the wall of the cavity, especially in CVM (**Fig. 23**). The vessel density and the Doppler shift

are low. Sometimes, a high RI is seen, indicating a normal arterial vessel in the mass.

The dysplastic venous malformation consists of multiple varicose veins. On B-mode imaging multiple anechoic tubular, tortuous channels infiltrating the subcutaneous fat, muscles, tendons, or other tissues are observed. Doppler interrogation reveals slow venous flow (**Fig. 24**).

Capillary Malformations

Capillary malformations are intradermal vascular anomalies.[33] They were previously named port-wine stains, but this obsolete denomination should not be used. Capillary malformations should not be confused with macular stains (nevus flammeus neonatorium)[34]; these pale pink macular stains are composed of ectatic dermal capillaries, occur in

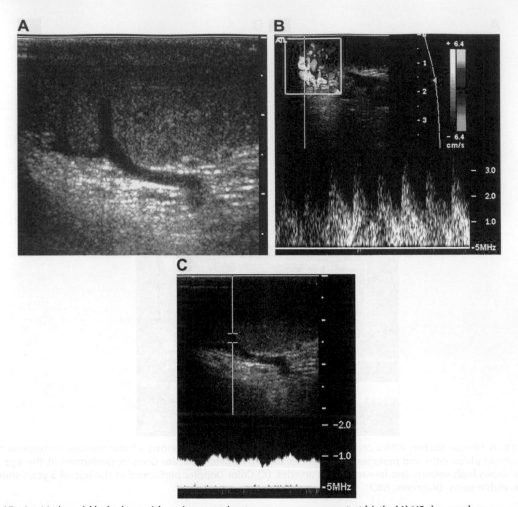

Fig. 15. An 11-day-old baby boy with a pigmented cutaneous mass present at birth. (*A*) US shows a homogeneous subcutaneous mass slightly echoic compared with fat. A large draining vein is present. (*B*) The lesion is hypervascular with arteries of high velocity and low resistance, and looks like a typical hemangioma. (*C*) The large vessel corresponds to a slightly pulsatile vein. Diagnosis: RICH.

35% to 50% of newborns, and usually regress. Capillary malformations are pink and flat at birth, with irregular borders. They usually involve the face but can occur anywhere on the body. It is important to exclude complex anomalies that can be associated with capillary malformations such as Sturge-Weber, Klippel-Trénaunay, Parkes Weber, Cobb, and Proteus syndromes, for which imaging studies are required.[2,35,36]

MRI is the imaging modality of choice for these syndromes. However, US can be useful in some indications. In the presence of a capillary malformation close to the midline of the spine in a newborn, a US examination of the spinal canal is indicated to exclude a tethered cord and dysraphism. Before laser treatment, it is important to look for an underlying AVM that can mimic a cutaneous capillary malformation.

Capillary malformations causing little aesthetic prejudice can be treated conservatively. If treatment is required, pulsed dye laser is the treatment of choice.

Lymphatic Malformations

Confusing terms are seen in the literature such as cystic hygroma or lymphangioma.[1] The

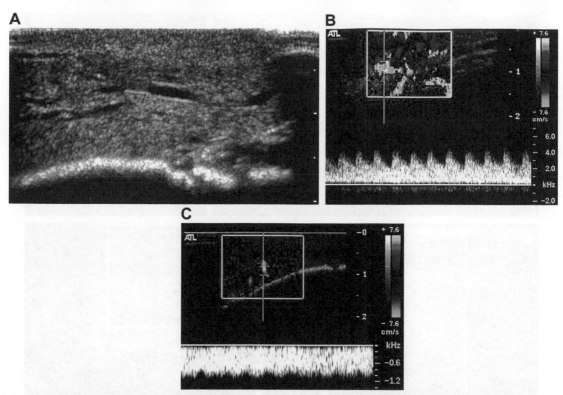

Fig. 16. An 8-day-old girl with a subcutaneous mass. (*A*) US shows a superficially located homogeneous mass containing dilated vessels. (*B*) The mass is hypervascular. High velocity and low resistance arteries are numerous. (*C*) The detection of pulsatile veins confirms the presence of abnormal arteriovenous communications. Diagnosis: RICH.

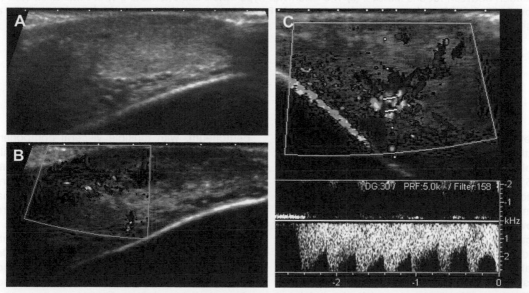

Fig. 17. A 3-year-old girl presenting with a progressive growing mass. (*A*) US shows a well-defined subcutaneous homogeneous mass. (*B*) Color Doppler shows that vessels are present mainly in the center of the mass. (*C*) High velocity arteries with low resistance are present in the center of the lesion. Diagnosis: hemangioendothelioma.

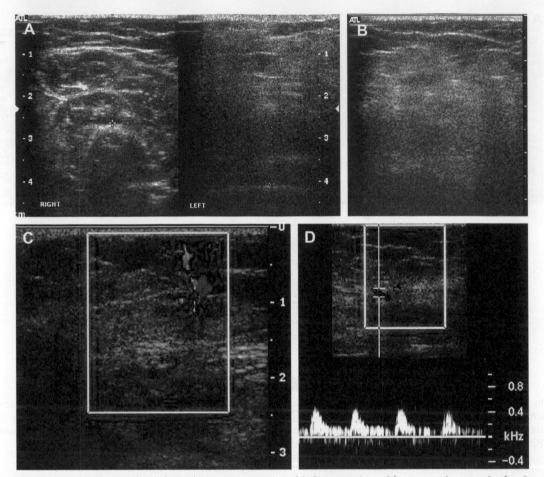

Fig. 18. A 4-year-old boy with a left thigh mass present since birth presenting with a recent increase in the size of the thigh. (*A*) Comparative US shows increased thickening of the soft tissues of the left thigh with loss of differentiation between fat and muscles. (*B*) The lesion was hyperechoic and attenuating with some small cysts (not shown). (*C*) Color Doppler reveals a few vessels. (*D*) Pulsed Doppler shows the arteries have low velocity and high resistance. Diagnosis: hemangioendothelioma.

preferred term to describe the underlying pathology is lymphatic malformation. Lymphatic malformations are usually present at birth (65%–75%), but sometimes they become evident only during childhood or adolescence.[37] Lymphatic malformations are localized or diffuse slow-flow soft-tissue lesions. The most common locations are the cervicofacial region, the axilla, and the upper chest. Three types of lymphatic malformation are described: macrocystic, microcystic, or mixed. The microcystic type is more infiltrative, with clear or hemorrhagic vesicles.[38] Diffuse lymphatic malformations can be seen within the thorax, the retroperitoneum, or the

peritoneum, with multiple visceral components. They can manifest by recurrent pleural effusion, pericardial effusion, and ascites. Involvement of the gastrointestinal tract, buttock, and anogenital area is frequently associated with limb lymphatic malformations. Chronic protein-losing enteropathy with hypoalbuminemia can occur when the gastrointestinal tract is involved. Involvement of an extremity can cause swelling and skeletal overgrowth. Gorham syndrome is a bone lymphatic malformation associated with bone degeneration and resorption.

Histologically, lymphatic malformations consist of chyle-filled cysts lined with endothelium.[39]

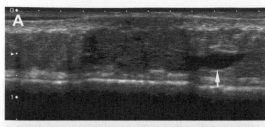

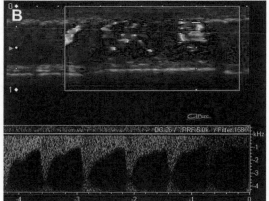

Fig. 19. A 4-year-old girl with a congenital lesion of the leg. (*A*) Homogeneous subcutaneous well-defined mass associated with a large irregular vessel (*arrow*). (*B*) Color Doppler shows a hypervascular lesion. High-velocity and low-resistance arteries are present. Diagnosis: tufted angioma (this type of lesion is rarely hypervascular).

Combined lymphatic venous malformations are common.

Sclerotherapy is the first choice for treatment of lymphatic malformation. Surgical approach is preferred in some institutions, particularly for microcystic lymphatic malformation.

US imaging

Gray-scale US permits lymphatic malformation characterization. Macrocystic lymphangiomas consist of a multiloculated cystic lesion (**Fig. 25**). Pure microcystic lesions are ill-defined and hyperechoic because of the numerous interfaces of the microcyst walls. Mixed lesions consist of cystic and solid components, related to the size of the cysts and their resulting US patterns (**Fig. 26**).

Color Doppler US shows vascular channels in the septa, including normal veins and arteries, as confirmed by spectral analysis (**Figs. 27** and **28**). In hemorrhagic or inflammatory complications, a fluid-fluid level can be observed in the cysts (**Fig. 29**).[14,40]

High-flow Malformations

AVM is defined as an abnormal connection between the arterial and venous system bypassing the capillary bed.[2] AVMs are congenital lesions, present at birth but not necessarily

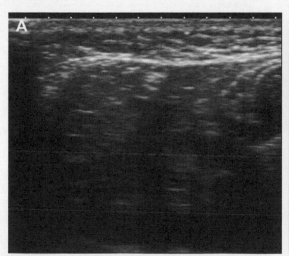

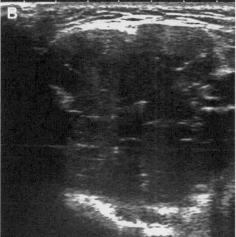

Fig. 20. A 14-year-old boy. A year previously, this boy presented with painful solid mass of the left cheek. The mass and pain regressed. However, painful increase of the mass occurred during effort or with flexion of the neck. Symptoms disappeared in dorsal decubitus position. (*A*) US performed in dorsal decubitus shows a well-delimited hypoechoic mass. (*B*) US performed with the head bowed shows an increase in volume of the venous lakes. Diagnosis: venous malformation.

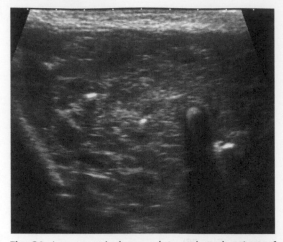

Fig. 21. Large cervical mass detected at the time of a third-trimester US. lymphatic malformation was suspected. After birth, US showed multiple small phleboliths (some with acoustic shadowing), suggesting venous malformation.

detectable clinically. They manifest in childhood or later, particularly during puberty. Trauma, biopsy, puberty, and pregnancy can trigger an acute exacerbation or flare-up.[41] They present clinically as a pulsatile mass, with a thrill, bruit, and occasionally local hyperthermia, skeletal overgrowth, trophic changes, congestive heart failure, and functional impairment. Cutaneous ischemia with ulceration or infection and hemorrhage are the most common complications. AVMs are usually isolated anomalies but can be part of a syndrome.

Treatment of AVMs is complex and should be reserved for symptomatic cases. The ideal treatment is selective embolization with or without surgical resection.

US imaging

On B-mode imaging, AVMs are poorly defined. The lesion consists of the juxtaposition of tortuous

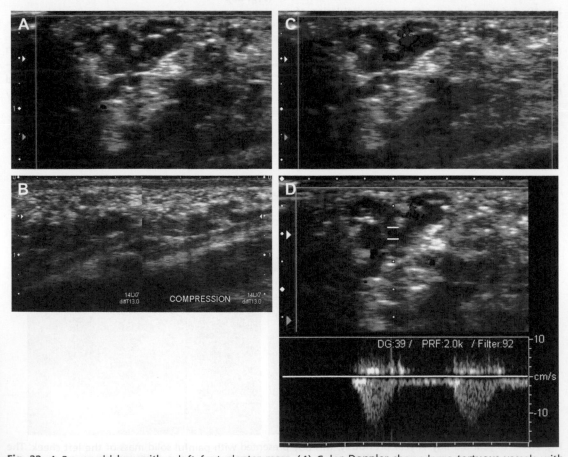

Fig. 22. A 3-year-old boy with a left foot plantar mass. (*A*) Color Doppler shows large tortuous vessels with internal echoes. (*B*) US shows the malformation is partially compressible. (*C*) After compression release, color Doppler shows some low-velocity flow. Phleboliths (with acoustic shadowing) are also present. (*D*) Only venous flow could be detected inside the abnormal vessels. Diagnosis: venous malformation.

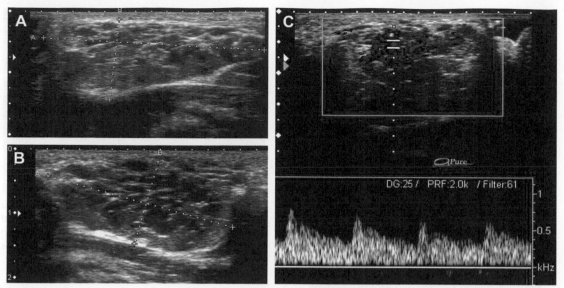

Fig. 23. (*A*) Well-delineated compressible mass. (*B*) Gray-scale US shows large vessels with low flow. (*C*) Low-resistance arteries are detected, suggesting the presence of a capillary component. Diagnosis: capillary venous malformation.

vessels. Sometimes the channels are seen within hyperechoic fat.[40]

Color Doppler and duplex US are instrumental for diagnosing AVMs. AVMs are characterized by multiple feeding arteries with increased diastolic flow and high-velocity venous return.[40] Unlike infantile hemangiomas, there is always arterialization of the venous flow in AVMs (**Figs. 30–32**).

SYNDROMES AND VASCULAR ANOMALIES
Syndromes with Vascular Stains and Slow-Flow Malformations

Klippel-Trénaunay syndrome
Klippel-Trénaunay syndrome is a capillary veno-lymphatic malformation with limb overgrowth. Clinical presentation is variable and depends on the predominance of abnormal lymphatic or

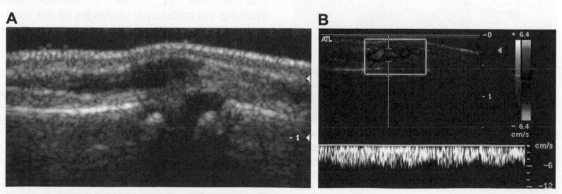

Fig. 24. A 6-year-old boy with abnormal pigmentation of the thumb since birth. Recently, the thumb has increased in volume. (*A*) US shows an irregular large compressible vessel in the soft tissues. (*B*) Pulsed Doppler shows typical venous flow. Diagnosis: venous malformation.

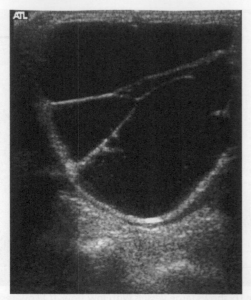

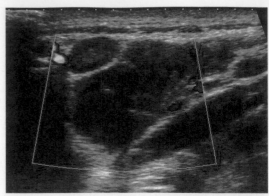

Fig. 27. A 16-year-old boy. Doppler US of the submaxillary region shows large cystic areas devoid of flow with delicate flow in the septae between the cysts. Diagnosis: macrocystic lymphatic malformation.

Fig. 25. Cervical cystic mass discovered during the third trimester of pregnancy. US performed in this 2-day-old girl confirms the diagnosis of cervical macrocystic lymphatic malformation.

venous vessels. This syndrome includes a dermal capillary stain associated with venous varicosities. These anomalous veins have deformed, insufficient, or absent valves. The pathognomonic marginal vein of Servelle is often identified in the subcutaneous fat of the lateral calf and thigh and can communicate with the deep venous system at various levels. Lymphedema can be associated, resulting from malformations and hypoplasia of the lymphatic vessels.

Blue rubber bleb nevus syndrome
This syndrome is characterized by multiple venous malformations of the skin with multiple gastrointestinal venous malformations. The gastrointestinal lesions can result in hemorrhage, intussuception, and volvulus. It is a sporadic disease, but familial cases have been reported.

Maffucci syndrome
Maffucci syndrome is a nonheritable syndrome that consists of diffuse enchondromatosis involving the metacarpal phalanges of the hands and feet associated with multiple venous or lymphatic malformations.

Proteus syndrome
This syndrome consists of multiple subcutaneous hamartomatous tumors, hemihypertrophy, pigmented nevi, gigantism involving the extremities (hand, foot), intra-abdominal lipomatosis, pachydermia, macrocephaly, bony exostoses, and lymphatic venous malformations.

Bannayan-Riley-Ruvalcaba syndrome
This syndrome is an autosomal dominant condition with a variable clinical phenotype. The

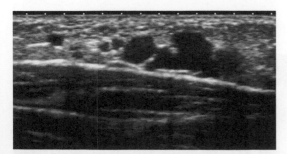

Fig. 26. A 5-year-old patient with a mass of the forearm present at birth. Fourteen days previously, the mass had become bluish. US shows the typical appearance of a mixed lymphatic malformation with noncompressible cysts associated with echoic thickening of the adjacent fat. Doppler US did not detect any flow inside the cysts, even with Valsalva maneuver. Diagnosis: mixed lymphatic malformation.

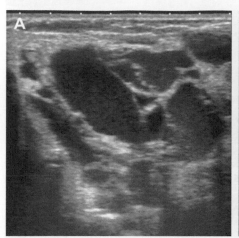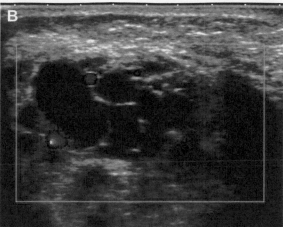

Fig. 28. A 1-month-old boy with a lateral cervical mass. Clinical diagnoses suggested teratoma. (*A*) US shows a heterogeneous soft uncompressible multicystic mass without calcification. (*B*) Doppler US reveals slow flow between the cysts. Diagnosis: macrocystic lymphatic malformation.

disorder is associated with PTEN gene mutation on chromosome 10q. Clinical features include macrocephaly, pseudopapilledema, pigmented maculas on the penis, gastrointestinal polyposis, visceral lipoma, thyroiditis, and capillary and combined malformations.

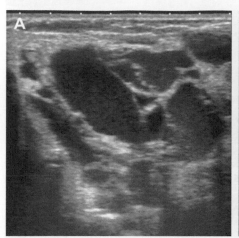

Fig. 29. A 4-year-old patient with a quiescent thoracic lymphatic malformation that suddenly increased. US shows echogenic fluid level corresponding to hemorrhage.

Glomovenous malformation
Glomovenous malformation is an autosomal-dominant condition, also known as glomangioma. It is characterized by multiple, often tender, blue nodular dermal lesions in the skin. Glomovenous malformation is multifocal and painful at palpation. US imaging features are similar to those of venous malformation with the exception that the lesion cannot be completely emptied by compression. The lesions are venous malformations with the presence of glomus cells (**Figs. 33** and **34**).

Syndromes with High-Flow Malformations

Parkes Weber syndrome
This syndrome combines AVFs, congenital varicose veins, and a cutaneous capillary malformation associated with limb hypertrophy.

Rendu-Osler-Weber syndrome (hereditary hemorrhagic telangiectasia)
The Rendu-Osler-Weber syndrome consists of diffuse mucosal telangiectasia involving the nasopharynx, the gastrointestinal tract, and sometimes the urinary and genital mucosa, AVFs and arterial aneurysms involving the pulmonary, hepatic, and digestive arteries.

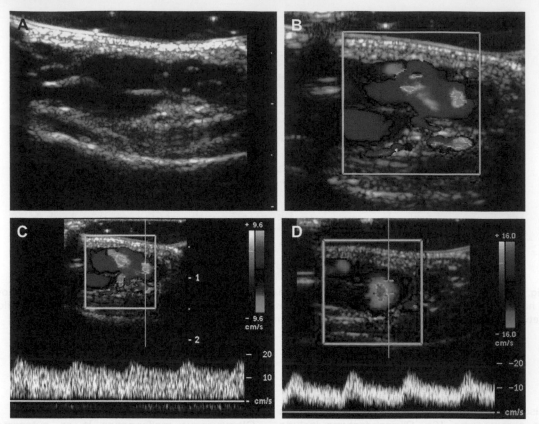

Fig. 30. A 16-year-old boy who developed collateral superficial vessels in his hand. (*A*) US shows isolated large vessels without associated abnormal tissue. (*B*) Color Doppler shows the vascular nature of the serpiginous anechoic structures. (*C*) High-velocity arteries with low resistance are present. (*D*) The enlarged veins have pulsatile flow. Diagnosis: AVM.

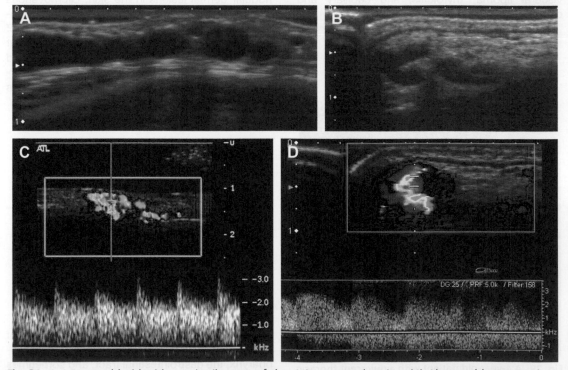

Fig. 31. A 4.5-year-old girl with a pulsatile mass of the right temporal region. (*A*) Abnormal large vessels are present in the subcutaneous tissue without any mass. (*B*) Large tortuous vessels are also detected deeply. (*C*) Doppler shows high-velocity and low-resistance arteries. (*D*) The abnormal vessels correspond to high-velocity arteries with low resistance and dilated pulsatile veins. Diagnosis: AVM.

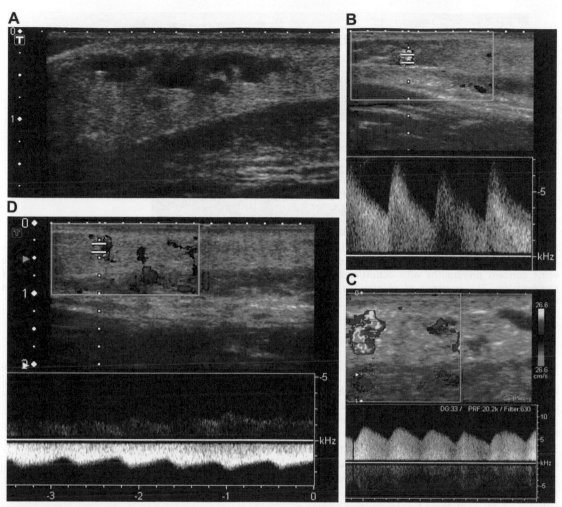

Fig. 32. A 3-year-old girl with a dorsal mass. (*A*) US reveals increased thickness of the subcutaneous fat around abnormal dilated vessels. (*B*) Doppler US shows high-velocity arteries with low RI. (*C*) Some dilated vessels are present, corresponding to high-flow pulsatile veins. (*D*) Doppler US shows pulsatile high-velocity venous flow typical of abnormal arteriovenous communications. Diagnosis: AVM.

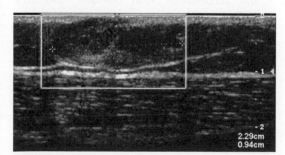

Fig. 33. A 10-year-old boy with multiple painful subcutaneous masses. On Doppler, the mass appears slightly compressible, heterogeneous, and with low vascularity. Diagnosis: glomovenous malformation.

Capillary malformation–AVM syndrome

Capillary malformation–AVM syndrome is a hereditary disorder characterized by cutaneous capillary malformation associated with AVM or AVF. Mutations in the RASA1 gene are reported in this condition.

Cobb syndrome

Cobb syndrome is a rare nonhereditary syndrome in which a cutaneous capillary malformation is associated with AVM of the spinal cord.

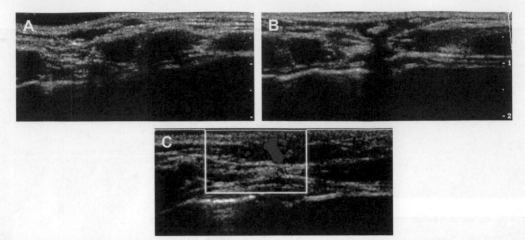

Fig. 34. A 3-year-old boy with a congenital vascular lesion of the anterior chest. The anomaly increased in size as the child grew. The child complained of pain. (*A*) Dilated subcutaneous veins observed at US. (*B*) Some veins contain phleboliths with acoustic shadowing. (*C*) On Doppler US, flow is disclosed after release of compression. The presence of phleboliths inside the abnormal veins is confirmed. Diagnosis: glomovenous malformation.

SUMMARY

Congenital vascular anomalies are frequently encountered in pediatrics, and may present as a dermatologic, orthopedic, ear, nose, and throat, hematologic, or visceral disorder. Proper nosology and terminology are paramount for effective multidisciplinary management. Imaging is useful for diagnosis at presentation and for follow-up. US including color and duplex Doppler is the best initial modality in children for recognizing hemangiomas and differentiating high-flow and slow-flow vascular anomalies.

REFERENCES

1. Morrison SC, Reid JR. Continuing problems with classifications of vascular malformations. Pediatr Radiol 2007;37(6):609.
2. Mulliken JB, Glowacki J. Hemangiomas and vascular malformations in infants and children: a classification based on endothelial characteristics. Plast Reconstr Surg 1982;69(3):412–22.
3. Mulliken JB, Fishman SJ, Burrows PE. Vascular anomalies. Curr Probl Surg 2000;37(8):517–84.
4. Dubois J, Patriquin HB, Garel L, et al. Soft-tissue hemangiomas in infants and children: diagnosis using Doppler sonography. AJR Am J Roentgenol 1998;171(1):247–52.
5. Chiller KG, Passaro D, Frieden IJ. Hemangiomas of infancy: clinical characteristics, morphologic subtypes, and their relationship to race, ethnicity, and sex. Arch Dermatol 2002;138(12):1567–76.

6. Frieden IJ, Haggstrom AN, Drolet BA, et al. Infantile hemangiomas: current knowledge, future directions. Proceedings of a research workshop on infantile hemangiomas. April 7-9, 2005. Bethesda, Maryland, USA. Pediatr Dermatol 2005;22(5): 383–406.
7. Haggstrom AN, Drolet BA, Baselga E, et al. Prospective study of infantile hemangiomas: clinical characteristics predicting complications and treatment. Pediatrics 2006;118(3):882–7.
8. Haggstrom AN, Lammer EJ, Scheiner RA, et al. Patterns of infantile hemangiomas: new clues to hemangioma pathogenesis and embryonic facial development. Pediatrics 2006;117(3):698–703.
9. Frieden IJ, Reese V, Cohen D. PHACE syndrome. The association of posterior fossa brain malformations, hemangiomas, arterial anomalies, coarctation of the aorta and cardiac defects, and eye abnormalities. Arch Dermatol 1996;132(3): 307–11.
10. Razon MJ, Kraling BM, Mulliken JB, et al. Increased apoptosis coincides with onset of involution in infantile hemangioma. Microcirculation 1998;5(2–3): 189–95.
11. Pollman MJ, Naumovski L, Gibbons GH. Vascular cell apoptosis: cell type-specific modulation by transforming growth factor-beta1 in endothelial cells versus smooth muscle cells. Circulation 1999; 99(15):2019–26.
12. North PE, Waner M, Mizeracki A, et al. GLUT1: a newly discovered immunohistochemical marker for juvenile hemangiomas. Hum Pathol 2000;31(1): 11–22.

13. Bakhach S, Grenier N, Berge J, et al. Color Doppler sonography of superficial capillary hemangiomas. J Radiol 2001;82(11):1613–9.

14. Paltiel HJ, Burrows PE, Kozakewich HPW, et al. Soft-tissue vascular anomalies: utility of US for diagnosis. Radiology 2000;214(3):747–54.

15. Boon LM, Enjolras O, Mulliken JB. Congenital hemangioma: evidence of accelerated involution. J Pediatr 1996;128(3):329–35.

16. North PE, Waner M, James CA, et al. Congenital nonprogressive hemangioma: a distinct clinicopathologic entity unlike infantile hemangioma. Arch Dermatol 2001;137(12):1607–20.

17. Mulliken JB, Enjolras O. Congenital hemangiomas and infantile hemangioma: missing links. J Am Acad Dermatol 2004;50(6):875–82.

18. Enjolras O, Mulliken JB, Boon LM, et al. Noninvoluting congenital hemangioma: a rare cutaneous vascular anomaly. Plast Reconstr Surg 2001; 107(7):1647–54.

19. Gorincour G, Kokta V, Rypens F, et al. Imaging characteristics of two subtypes of congenital hemangiomas: rapidly involuting congenital hemangiomas and non-involuting congenital hemangiomas. Pediatr Radiol 2005;35(12):1178–85.

20. Rogers M, Lam A, Fischer G. Sonographic findings in a series of rapidly involuting congenital hemangiomas (RICH). Pediatr Dermatol 2002;19(1):5–11.

21. Vin-Christian K, McCalmont TH, Frieden IJ. Kaposiform hemangioendothelioma. An aggressive, locally invasive vascular tumor that can mimic hemangioma of infancy. Arch Dermatol 1997;133(12):1573–8.

22. Enjolras O, Wassef M, Mazoyer E, et al. Infants with Kasabach-Merritt syndrome do not have "true" hemangiomas. J Pediatr 1997;130(4):631–40.

23. Sarkar M, Mulliken JB, Kozakewich HP, et al. Thrombocytopenic coagulopathy (Kasabach-Merritt phenomenon) is associated with Kaposiform hemangioendothelioma and not with common infantile hemangioma. Plast Reconstr Surg 1997;100(16): 1377–86.

24. Enjolras O, Mulliken JB, Wassef M, et al. Residual lesions after Kasabach-Merritt phenomenon in 41 patients. J Am Acad Dermatol 2000;42(2 Pt 1): 225–35.

25. Dubois J, Garel L, David M, et al. Vascular soft-tissue tumors in infancy: distinguishing features on Doppler sonography. AJR Am J Roentgenol 2002; 178(6):1541–5.

26. Abernethy LJ. Classification and imaging of vascular malformations in children. Eur Radiol 2003;13(11): 2483–97.

27. Trop I, Dubois J, Guibaud L, et al. Soft-tissue venous malformations in pediatric and young adult patients: diagnosis with Doppler US. Radiology 1999;212(3): 841–5.

28. Wirth GA, Sundine MJ. Slow-flow vascular malformations. Clin Pediatr (Phila) 2007;46(2):109–20.

29. Mazoyer E, Enjolras O, Laurian C, et al. Coagulation abnormalities associated with extensive venous malformations of the limbs: differentiation from Kasabach-Merritt syndrome. Clin Lab Haematol 2002; 24(4):243–51.

30. Boon LM, Mulliken JB, Vikkula M, et al. Assignment of a locus for dominantly inherited venous malformations to chromosome 9p. Hum Mol Genet 1994;3(9): 1583–7.

31. Vikkula M, Boone LM, Carraway KL 3rd, et al. Vascular dysmorphogenesis caused by activating mutation in the receptor tyrosine kinase TIE2. Cell 1996;87(7):1181–90.

32. Boon LM, Brouillard P, Irrthum A, et al. A gene for inherited cutaneous venous anomalies ("glomangiomas") localizes to chromosome 1p21–22. Am J Hum Genet 1999;65(1):125–33.

33. Spring MA, Bentz ML. Cutaneous vascular lesions. Clin Plast Surg 2005;32(2):171–86.

34. Tan KL. Nevus flammeus of the nape, glabella and eyelids. A clinical study of frequency, racial distribution, and association with congenital anomalies. Clin Pediatr (Phila) 1972;11(2):112–8.

35. Esterly NB. Cutaneous hemangiomas, vascular stains and malformations, and associated syndromes. Curr Probl Pediatr 1996;26(1):3–39.

36. Marler JJ, Mulliken JB. Current management of hemangiomas and vascular malformations. Clin Plast Surg 2005;32(1):99–116.

37. Garzon MC, Huang JT, Enjolras O, et al. Vascular malformations: part I. J Am Acad Dermatol 2007; 56(3):353–70.

38. Enjolras O. Classification and management of the various superficial vascular anomalies: hemangiomas and vascular malformations. J Dermatol 1997;24(11):701–10.

39. Koeller KK, Alamo L, Adair CF, et al. Congenital cystic masses of the neck: radiologic-pathologic correlation. Radiographics 1999;19(1):121–46.

40. Dubois J, Garel L, Grignon A, et al. Imaging of hemangiomas and vascular malformations in children. Acad Radiol 1998;5(5):390–400.

41. Kohout MP, Hansen M, Pribaz JJ, et al. Arteriovenous malformations of the head and neck: natural history and management. Plast Reconstr Surg 1998;102(3):643–54.

Modern Head Ultrasound: Normal Anatomy, Variants, and Pitfalls That May Simulate Disease

Kay North, DO*, Lisa H. Lowe, MD

KEYWORDS

- Normal • Ultrasound • Anatomy • Neonatal
- Head • Brain

The first ultrasound imaging of the head, in 1955, used A-mode imaging techniques to obtain crude pictures to estimate ventricular size.[1] Since then, advances in equipment and techniques have made ultrasound a highly accurate method for intracranial evaluation. While ultrasound has its limitations, recent studies comparing magnetic resonance imaging and computed tomography to careful head sonogram have shown that, for detecting abnormalities, ultrasound offers the accuracy required to make an initial diagnosis and guide management.[2] Ultrasound has the benefit of being portable, which means it may be performed at the bedside of unstable infants who cannot safely be brought to radiology for other neuroimaging. In addition, ultrasound does not expose the infant to radiation and is less expensive than other imaging modalities.

OVERVIEW OF CRANIAL ULTRASOUND TECHNIQUE

Gray-scale head ultrasound is performed first via the anterior fontanelle in the coronal plane, after which the transducer is turned 90° and additional images are obtained in the sagittal and parasagittal planes.[3] Second, routine imaging of the posterior fossa through the posterolateral fontanelle (also called the mastoid fontanelle) is the current standard of care, but it is a relatively new

technique and is not always employed. Third, screening Doppler ultrasound of the intracranial vasculature can be routinely obtained from the anterior fontanelle or the transtemporal approach. Ideally, screening Doppler during infant head ultrasound includes a spectral tracing from the right and left middle cerebral arteries and a midline sagittal venous image, including the sagittal sinus and vein of Galen.

Typically six or more coronal images are taken, with the first image (most anterior) obtained through the frontal lobes just anterior to the frontal horns and the sixth (most posterior) obtained through the occipital lobes just posterior to the trigone of the lateral ventricles.[4] At least five images are obtained in the sagittal plane. The first image performed is midline. A good midline image is obtained when both the vermis and corpus callosum are clearly seen on the image. Next, two to three images each of the right and left parasagittal brain are obtained at graded increments extending from just off midline (near the caudothalamic groove) to the Sylvian fissures.[4] A single image of the right and left posterior fossa structures is obtained through both mastoid fontanelles. Structures identified on the mastoid (posterolateral fontanelle) views include the cerebellum, cerebellar vermis, fourth ventricle, and cisterna magna. Screening head ultrasound Doppler images are obtained via the anterior fontanelle or transtemporal (anterolateral fontanelle)

Department of Radiology, University of Missouri-Kansas City School of Medicine, Children's Mercy Hospitals and Clinics, 2401 Gillham Road, Kansas City, MO 64108, USA
* Corresponding author.
E-mail address: klnorth@cmh.edu (K. North).

Ultrasound Clin 4 (2009) 497–512
doi:10.1016/j.cult.2009.11.003
1556-858X/09/$ – see front matter © 2009 Elsevier Inc. All rights reserved.

ultrasound.theclinics.com

approach. Vascular structures can be screened for patency and resistance, providing information about intracranial blood flow. Routine screening measurements include the peak systolic velocity, end diastolic velocity, and resistive index (RI).[5]

Interpretation of Modern Cranial Ultrasound

Today's savvy radiologist uses all imaging techniques available to do far more than was possible in the past. Beyond understanding basic cranial ultrasound anatomy, one must be familiar with the various fontanelles that may be used for imaging, the normal echogenicity of anatomic structures throughout the brain, normal routine Doppler screening, and high-resolution linear imaging.

To obtain high-quality head ultrasound images, it is essential to maintain side-to-side symmetry. Regarding image echogenicity, a basic rule is that gray matter structures tend to be hypoechoic and of similar echogenicity, regardless of their location (eg, gray matter of the cerebral cortex or basal ganglia). Similarly, white matter structures tend be of increased echogenicity and similar to one another.

Throughout the brain, the distinct echogenic pia matter can be seen as a well-defined thin layer covering the hypoechoic superficial gray matter cortex (Fig. 1). Loss of this layer may indicate edema, ischemia, or infarction (Fig. 2). Because infants often have symmetric abnormalities involving the basal ganglia, it is important to carefully analyze the echogenicity of gray versus white matter structures to avoid missing symmetric abnormalities. This extra care is especially important in images involving the thalami. The thalami,

being mostly gray matter, are normally equal in echogenicity to the adjacent basal ganglia gray matter. However, if the thalamus resembles the echogenicity of the adjacent white matter, it is abnormal and may indicate thalamic edema/ischemia or infarction, which can occur with severe hypoxic ischemic injury (Fig. 3).[6]

CRANIAL ULTRASOUND ANATOMY
Coronal Anatomy

Beginning in the anterior coronal plane, the frontal lobes and orbital cones are seen on the first image (Fig. 4). The interhemispheric fissure contains the falx cerebri, it is the most midline structure, and is highly echogenic.[7]

Progressing posteriorly, the second coronal image shows the frontal horns of the lateral ventricles as paired paramedian, anechoic structures filled with cerebral spinal fluid (CSF) (Fig. 5).[3] The caudate heads form the lateral walls of the lateral ventricles. The corpus callosum is a linear hypoechoic structure with a well-defined tram track–like echogenic superior and inferior border that crosses the midline and serves as the roof of the lateral ventricles. The corpus callosum is the major pathway for tracts crossing from one hemisphere to the other and the thickness reflects the volume of periventricular white matter. The medial walls of the lateral ventricles are formed by the cavum septum pellicidum.[3] Immediately above the corpus callosum are the cingulate gyrus and pericallosal sulcus. Normal gyri are composed of superficial hypoechoic gray matter cortex, which overlies the deeper hyperechoic subcortical white matter. The putamen and globus pallidus (lentiform nuclei) are both gray matter structures

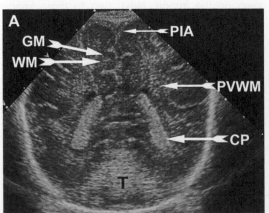
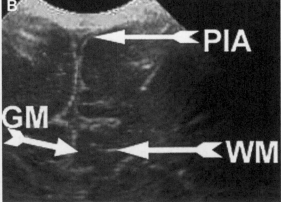

Fig. 1. Normal cortex in a term infant. (A and B) Coronal images of the brain demonstrate the layers of the cortex, including the superficial linear hyperechoic pia matter (PIA), which overlies the hypoechoic gray matter (GM), which overlies the hyperechoic subcortical white matter (WM) and periventricular white matter (PVWM). Also noted are the choroid plexus (CP) and the tentorium cerebelli (T).

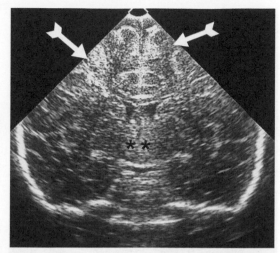

Fig. 2. Loss of cortical gray-white differentiation in a term infant with hypoxic ischemic brain injury due to sepsis. Coronal sonogram reveals poor visualization of the normal layers of the cortex (*arrows*). The medial thalami are hyperechoic bilaterally (*asterisks*).

Fig. 4. Normal cranial ultrasound through the frontal lobes in a term infant. Coronal image shows the midline interhemispheric fissure (IF), which contains the echogenic falx cerebri. The echogenic floor of the anterior cranial fossa is seen just below the frontal lobes (FL) and above the orbital cones (OC).

located lateral and inferior to the caudate nucleus. Echogenic Y-shaped Sylvian fissures are located laterally and serve to divide the temporal from the frontal lobes.[3] On real-time imaging, the vascular structures of the circle of Willis are seen in the suprasellar cistern and the middle cerebral

arteries can be seen pulsating within the Sylvain fissures.

The third image, obtained at the level of the foramina of Monro, shows that the caudate nuclei serve as the lateral walls of the ventricular system, the corpus callosum serves as the roof, and the septum pellicudum serves as the medial wall (**Fig. 6**). On real-time imaging, the pericallosal arteries can be seen pulsating just superior to the hypoechoic corpus callosum.[1] The third ventricle, which is variably visualized, is a thin midline anechoic structure located between the thalami. The pons and medulla are midline brainstem structures located inferior to the third ventricle.[3]

The fourth image obtained is just posterior to the third ventricle (**Fig. 7**). The thalami border the lateral ventricles inferiorly.[3] The echogenic choroid plexus appears as three echogenic foci in the roof of the third ventricle and along the floors of the lateral ventricles.[3,4] The hyperechoic tentorium cerebelli is located above the relatively hypoechoic cerebellar hemispheres.[3] The cerebral peduncles are hypoechoic structures located inferior to the thalami.[3]

The fifth image is performed through the echogenic quadrigeminal plate cistern (**Fig. 8**).[3] The temporal horns of the lateral ventricles and sometimes the mammillary bodies may be visualized at this level.[3] The echogenic tentorium cerebelli demarcates the superior aspect of the posterior fossa.[7] The cerebellar vermis is an echogenic midline structure with the cisterna magna located more posterior and inferior.[3]

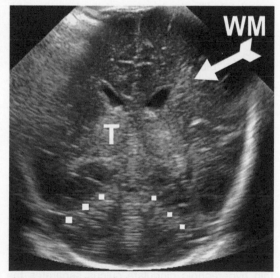

Fig. 3. Hyperechoic thalami due to hypoxic ischemic deep nuclear injury in an acidotic term infant. Coronal ultrasound shows increased echogenicity of the thalami (T), which are normally hypoechoic in comparison to the adjacent deep white matter (WM) and tentorium cerebelli (*dots*).

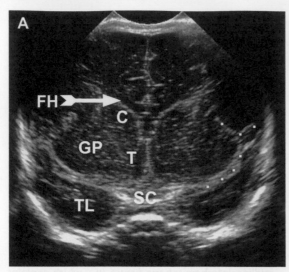

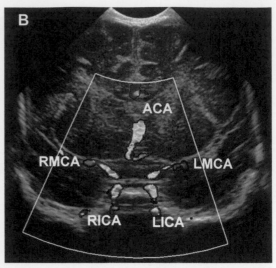

Fig. 5. Normal cranial ultrasound through the frontal horns and circle of Willis in a term infant. (*A*) Coronal gray-scale image reveals the caudate (C) nuclei, the frontal horns (FH), and globus pallidus (GP). Note the thalamus (T), which is just below and similar in echogenicity to the caudate nuclei. Dots indicate the echogenic Y-shaped Sylvian fissures. Also noted are the temporal lobes (TL) and the suprasellar cistern (SC), which is where the circle of Willis is located. (*B*) Coronal Doppler image demonstrates the vessels of the circle of Willis, including the right internal carotid artery (RICA), the left internal carotid artery (LICA), the middle cerebral artery (RMCA), the left middle cerebral artery (LMCA), and the anterior cerebral arteries (ACA).

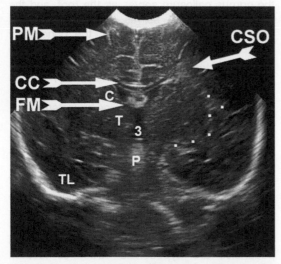

Fig. 6. Normal cranial ultrasound through the foramina of Monro and the third ventricle in a term infant. Coronal image identifies the midline hypoechoic corpus callosum (CC), which is demarcated by thin echogenic lines along the superior and inferior borders. The third ventricle (3) is variably visualized as a midline anechoic space below the septum pellucidum. Also noted are the echogenic belly of the pons (P), temporal lobes (TL), caudate nucleus (C), thalamus (T), centrum semiovale (CSO), foramen of Monro (FM), Sylvian fissures (*dots*), and pia matter (PM).

Continuing posteriorly, the sixth image is obtained at the level of the lateral ventricle trigones (**Fig. 9**). The ventricles diverge laterally from their more anterior midline location within the frontal lobes.[1,3] The glomus of the choroid plexus is a highly echogenic structure that nearly completely fills the trigones of the lateral ventricles. The deep periventricular white matter runs parallel to the lateral ventricles, is slightly hyperechoic, and is referred to as the periventricular "halo" or "blush."[3,8] In general, the periventricular halo is normal if the echogenicity is less than that of the adjacent choroid plexus.[3]

The seventh, or final, image is obtained posterior to the lateral ventricle trigones through the convexities of the cerebral hemispheres (**Fig. 10**). The interhemispheric fissure is well visualized[3]

Sagittal Anatomy

In the midline, the corpus callosum is seen as a hypoechoic C-shaped structure with a well-defined tram track–like echogenic superior and inferior border (**Fig. 11**). The cingulate gyrus is seen arching above the corpus callosum and the thin hyperechoic cingulate sulcus separates the cingulate gyrus from the more superficial gyri.[3] The cavum septum pellicidum is a fluid-filled structure below the corpus callosum and above the third ventricle.[3] The third and fourth ventricles are located in the midline.[3] Echogenic choroid plexus

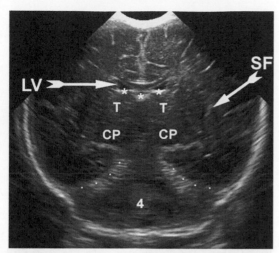

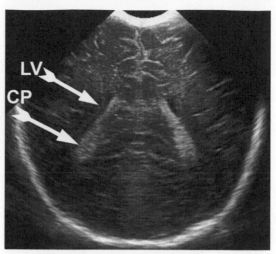

Fig. 7. Normal cranial ultrasound through the cerebral peduncles in a term infant. Coronal image shows the hyperechoic tentorium cerebelli (*dots*), which separate the supratentorial brain from the posterior fossa. Also noted are the hypoechoic cerebral peduncles (CP), thalami (T), the lateral ventricles (LV), the Sylvian fissures (SF), the fourth ventricles (4), and the echogenic choroid plexus along the floor of the lateral and roof of the third ventricles, giving the appearance of three dots (*asterisks*).

Fig. 9. Normal cranial ultrasound through the lateral ventricles in a term infant. Coronal image demonstrates the echogenic choroid plexus (CP) within the lateral ventricle (LV). The periventricular halo is seen as a slight hyperechogenicity within the deep white matter.

is seen lining the roof of the third ventricle and should not be mistaken for intraventricular hemorrhage or a germinal matrix bleed, the latter of which is seen on the parasagittal images at the caudothalamic grooves.[3] The cerebral aqueduct

of Sylvius extends from the posterior margin of the third ventricle through the hypoechoic midbrain,[1] and is the pathway of CSF flow from the third ventricle to the fourth ventricle. The belly of the pons, which contains many white matter tracts, is echogenic compared with the hypoechoic midbrain and dorsal aspect of the brainstem.[9] The cisterna magna is a normal anechoic fluid-containing structure located between the

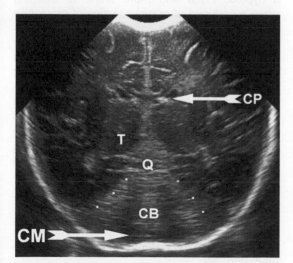

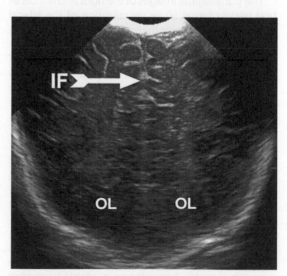

Fig. 8. Normal cranial ultrasound through the quadrigeminal plate cistern in a term infant. Coronal image reveals the quadrigeminal plate cistern (Q), the symmetric hypoechoic cerebellar hemispheres (CB), the cisterna magna (CM), the choroid plexus (CP) in the lateral ventricle, the thalamus (T), and tentorium cerebelli (*dots*).

Fig. 10. Normal cranial ultrasound through the cerebral convexities in a term infant. Coronal image identifies the interhemispheric fissure (IF) and the occipital lobes (OL).

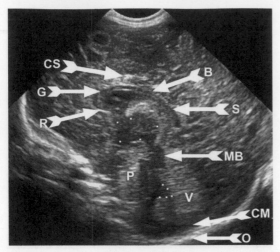

Fig. 11. Normal midline cranial ultrasound in a term infant. Sagittal image shows the genu (G), body (B), splenium (S), and rostrum (R) of the corpus callosum. Also noted are the cingulate sulcus (CS), echogenic belly of pons (P), echogenic kidney bean– or Pac-Man–shaped vermis (V) just above the cisterna magna (CM), the occipital bone (O), and the hypoechoic midbrain (MB). Dots outline the third and fourth ventricles.

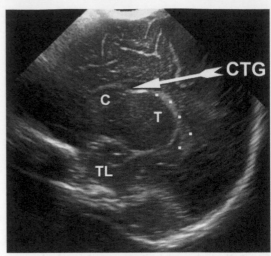

Fig. 12. Normal parasagittal cranial ultrasound in a term infant. Image angled through the lateral ventricle demonstrates the caudothalamic grove (CTG), caudate nucleus (C), thalamus (T), and temporal lobe (TL). Dots outline the comma-shaped intraventricular choroid plexus.

vermis and the occipital bone.[3] On real-time Doppler imaging, many arterial structures, such as the anterior cerebral arteries, may be visualized pulsating in their expected locations.[1,7] The occipital bone demarcates the posterior aspect of the foramen magnum at the inferior margin of the posterior fossa.[1]

The parasagittal images of the right and left cerebral hemispheres allow visualization of the lateral ventricles. The caudothalamic groove divides the caudate nucleus from the thalamus and demarcates the anterior attachment of the choroid plexus. The caudate nucleus is similar to or slightly more echogenic than the adjacent thalamus (Fig. 12).[3] Evaluation of the gray-white junction is performed on all images in addition to assessment of the sulci and gyri for uniform size and shape.

The germinal matrix, a zone of cells that eventually give rise to the neurons and glia of the brain, is a normal structure in premature infants.[6] Although the normal germinal matrix cannot be visualized with ultrasound, understanding its development and pathophysiology are important to the interpretation of cranial ultrasound. The normal fetal periventricular germinal matrix gradually involutes before 34 weeks' gestation, so it is rare to have a germinal matrix hemorrhage in infants born after this time.[6] In premature infants, residual germinal matrix is found at the caudothalamic groove, and is therefore the most common location for

germinal matrix hemorrhages. Anatomically, the germinal matrix is composed of capillaries lined by simple endothelium. Compared to other vessels in the fetal brain, these capillaries are larger, more numerous, and have an increased number of mitochondria. These capillaries thus have higher oxidative requirements.[6] The aforementioned characteristics of the germinal matrix cause it to be easily damaged when exposed to a hypoxic insult and more prone to bleeding when reperfused after resuscitation of premature infants.[6]

Parasagittal images obtained more laterally show the occipital and temporal horns of the lateral ventricles as CSF- and choroid plexus–containing structures (Fig. 13). The choroid plexus is highly echogenic and extends from the third ventricle through the foramina of Monro into the lateral ventricles.[3] It tapers gradually as it courses toward its attachment at the caudothalamic groove, although occasional lobulation can be seen as a normal variant.[3,7] The size of the lateral ventricles varies from a tiny slitlike structure to a moderate-size CSF-filled crescentaric collection.[3]

The final parasagittal image of the right and left cerebral hemispheres is obtained through the lateral aspect of the thalamus and peripheral cerebrum (Fig. 14).

Posterior Fossa Anatomy

Posterior fossa views can assess the radiating surface folds (folia) of the cerebellum, the cisterna

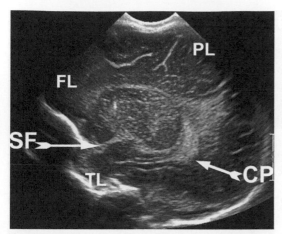

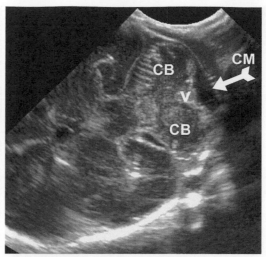

Fig. 13. Normal parasagittal cranial ultrasound in a term infant. Image through the lateral ventricle reveals the echogenic choroid plexus (CP) and Sylvian fissure (SF). Also identified are the frontal lobe (FL), temporal lobe (TL), and parietal lobe (PL). Incidentally noted is linear echogenicity along the anterior margin of the thalamus due to lenticulostriate vasculopathy.

Fig. 15. Normal posterior fossa ultrasound in a term infant. Image performed via the mastoid fontanelle shows the cerebellar hemispheres (CB), cisterna magna (CM), cerebellar vermis (V).

magna, and the fourth ventricle for normal appearance and size (**Fig. 15**). Because recent studies have shown a significant improvement in detecting posterior fossa hemorrhages, these views are now the standard of care for imaging the anatomic structures of the hindbrain (**Fig. 16**). Color Doppler interrogation of the posterior circulation, transverse sinus, and straight sinus can also be performed if needed.[3]

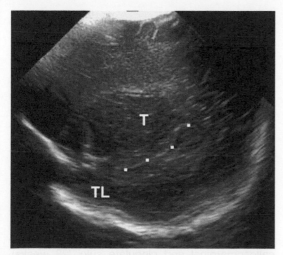

Fig. 14. Normal parasagittal cranial ultrasound in a term infant. Image obtained lateral to the lateral ventricle demonstrates the cerebral cortex. Noted are the thalamus (T), temporal lobe (TL), and Sylvian fissure (*dots*).

Color and Spectral Doppler Anatomy

Color Doppler images of the circle of Willis are part of the routine screening images obtained in the coronal plane via the anterior fontanelle (see **Fig. 5**), or in the axial plane via the transtemporal approach. In deciding which fontanelle to use during screening cranial ultrasound, clinicians choose according to the vessel they want to interrogate or, more commonly, they choose the fontanelle that is most convenient.[4] For routine screening head ultrasound, the anterior fontanelle is usually the most convenient and is adequate, but for a more detailed evaluation of the circle of Willis, the transtemporal approach is best.

Although a detailed discussion of transcranial Doppler applications is beyond the scope of this article, it is important to be familiar with the basics of cranial Doppler ultrasound to perform proper screening. Normal arterial Doppler spectra obtained from the circle of Willis show antegrade flow throughout the cardiac cycle with a rapid upstroke during systole and a gradual downstroke during diastole (**Fig. 17**).[4] The RI (ie, [systolic velocity − diastolic velocity] ÷ systolic velocity[10]) can be used to assess for alterations in intracranial blood flow dynamics.[11] Variations in flow velocity, blood volume, or vascular resistance will be reflected in the RI values.[11] The normal RI gradually decreases with age (**Table 1**).[5,12,13] The gradual decrease in RI is thought to be due to increasing diastolic flow velocities, changes in peripheral cerebrovascular

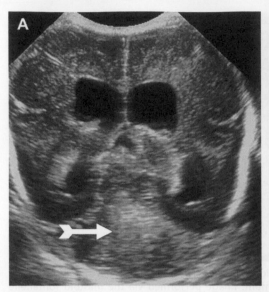
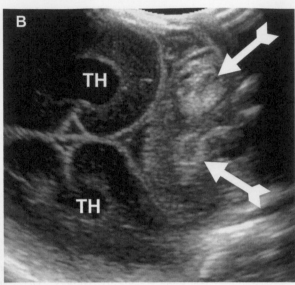

Fig. 16. Posterior fossa hemorrhage in a premature infant. (*A*) Coronal ultrasound image demonstrates a hyperechoic region in the left cerebellum (*arrow*). Also seen is posthemorrhagic hydrocephalus. (*B*) Posterior fossa view eloquently confirms the cerebellar hemorrhage (*arrows*). Also labeled are the temporal horns of lateral ventricles (TH).

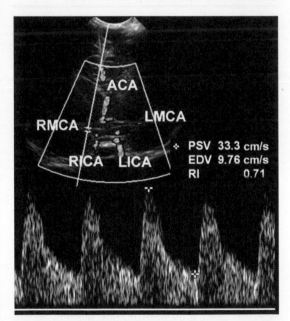

Fig. 17. Normal cranial ultrasound with color Doppler and spectral tracing in a term infant. Labeled vessels on the color image include the anterior cerebral arteries (ACA), left middle cerebral artery (LMCA), right middle cerebral arteries (RMCA), right internal carotid artery (RICA), and left internal carotid arteries (LICA). Note the normal rapid upstroke of systole and gradual downstroke of diastole, both of which are above the baseline throughout the cardiac cycle. A normal RI of 0.71 is present. PSV, peak systolic velocity; EDV, end-diastolic velocity.

circulation, and the switch from fetal to newborn circulation, including closure of a ductus arteriosus.[4] Note that the RI is not reliable in the setting of cardiac disease. For further information on the varied applications of transcranial Doppler in infants and children, see the article by Bulas and colleagues elsewhere in this issue.

NORMAL VARIANTS AND PITFALLS THAT MAY SIMULATE DISEASE
Immature Sulcation of the Premature Infant

Because the appearance of the normal infant brain changes significantly from 24 to 40 weeks of age, knowledge of the normal appearance at various stages of development is important. In premature infants under 24 weeks of age, the cerebral cortex has a smooth appearance with formation of only the Sylvian fissures.[4] Because of this, radiologists must avoid the pitfall of a diagnosis of lissencephaly before 24 weeks of gestational age. Specific sulci become visible as infants mature. These sulci include the parieto-occipital fissure (24 weeks), the callosomarginal and cingulate sulci (28 weeks), and branches arising from the cingulate sulcus (30 weeks) (**Figs. 18** and **19**).[4] As infants mature from 30 to 40 weeks, sulci gradually branch, becoming more complex.[4]

Table 1 Normal RIs by age	
Age	Normal RI
Premature infant	0.77
Term infant	0.65–0.75
Child>2 y	0.43–0.58

Persistent Fetal Ventricles: Cavum Septum Pellucidum, Cavum Vergae, and Velum Interpositum

The cavum septum pellucidum, cavum vergae, and velum interpositum are normal fetal ventricles that close from posterior to anterior starting at about 6 months of gestational age. When the leaves of the cavum septum pellucidum fail to fuse, a CSF-filled midline structure can remain.[14] Persistent fetal ventricles can be distinguished by their characteristic location. The cavum septum pellucidum, located between the frontal horns of the lateral ventricle, is the most anterior of these structures (**Fig. 20**).[14] Extension of the cavum septum pellucidum posterior to the fornices is termed *cavum septum pellucidum et vergae* or simply *cavum vergae*.[14,15] Further posterior extension of the fetal cavum into the pineal region is termed *cavum velum interpositum* or simply *velum interpositum*. Care must be taken not to mistake the cavum velum interpositum for other pineal region cystic structures, such as

a congenital cyst or vein of Galen malformation (**Fig. 21**).[14,16]

By 38 to 40 weeks' gestation, 97% of the cavum vergae have closed. The cavum septum pellucidum closes in 85% of infants by 3 to 6 months of age.[4] Occasionally, normal fetal ventricles may persist into adulthood and are of no clinical significance. Given the direction of closure, a cavum vergae or cavum velum interpositum is rarely seen in the absence of a cavum septum pellucidum.[17]

Mega Cisterna Magna

The normal cisterna magna measures 3 to 8 mm in the sagittal plane from the posterior lip of the foramen magnum to the caudal margin of the inferior vermis. In the axial plane, it normally measures less than 8 mm (**Fig. 22**).[14,18] If the cisterna magna measures more than 8 mm, the term *mega cisterna magna* is applied. Although a mega cisterna magna may appear alarming at first glance, it is a normal variant seen in 1% of postnatally imaged brains and is of no clinical significance.[14,19] It can be distinguished by its typical size, midline retrocerebellar location, and lack of mass effect (**Fig. 23**). Other common retrocerebellar posterior fossa cysts include arachnoid cysts (benign, congenital, typically clinically insignificant, CSF-containing cysts with mass effect), and Dandy-Walker malformations (complete or total absence of the vermis associated with an enlarged posterior fossa).[14]

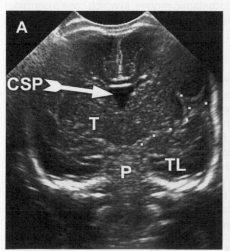
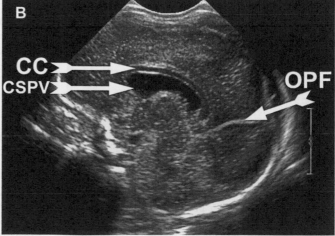

Fig. 18. Normal cranial ultrasound in a premature infant born at 26 weeks gestational age. (*A*) Coronal and (*B*) sagittal images show smooth cortex with only formation of the Sylvian fissures (*dots*). Also noted are the midline fluid-filled cavum septum pellucidum (CSP), cavum septum pellucidum et verge (CSPV), pons (P), temporal lobes (TL), thalamus (T), occipital parietal fissure (OPF), and corpus callosum (CC).

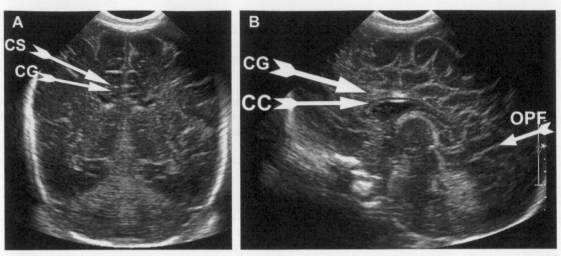

Fig. 19. Normal cranial ultrasound in a premature infant born at 30 weeks gestational age. (*A*) Coronal and (*B*) sagittal images reveal complex gyral and sulcal pattern. Labeled structures include the cingulate sulcus (CS), cingulate gyrus (CG), corpus callosum (CC), and occipital parietal fissure (OPF).

Asymmetric Ventricular Size

The ventricles are considered normal in size if they measure less than 10 mm in transverse diameter.[20] Mild ventriculomegaly is diagnosed when the ventricles measure from 10 to 12 mm.[20] The lateral ventricles of most infants (60% term and 30% premature) measure less than 2 to 3 mm in diameter.[3,21] In general, the lateral ventricles are largest in premature infants and become progressively smaller as the infant matures.[3] In 20% to

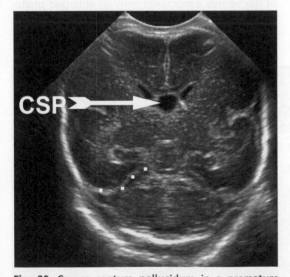

Fig. 20. Cavum septum pellucidum in a premature infant born at 29 weeks gestational age. The normal fetal cavum septum pellucidum (CSP) is seen between the frontal horns immediately below the corpus callosum and above, but separate from, the third ventricle. Dots indicate the tentorium cerebelli. Note the limited sulcation of the 29-week-premature infant brain.

40% of infants, some degree of lateral ventricle asymmetry can be seen.[3,21,22] The occipital horns are usually larger than the frontal horns and the left ventricle is more often larger than the right.[3,22] Finally, ventricular size can fluctuate with positioning of the patient, with the down-side ventricle smaller than the up-side ventricle (**Fig. 24**).[3,23]

Choroid Plexus Variants

The choroid plexus typically fills the trigones of lateral ventricles, gradually tapering anteriorly and posteriorly to a thin, smooth attachment.[3] It extends from the roof of the third ventricle through the foramina of Monro into the lateral ventricles.[3] The choroid plexus should not extend anterior to the caudothalamic groove, in which case a germinal matrix hemorrhage should be considered, or into occipital horns of the lateral ventricles, which may indicate intraventricular hemorrhage.[3,9] The glomus, the largest portion of the choroid plexus located within the ventricular atria, may have a variable lobular or bulbous appearance (**Fig. 25**).[3,24] Normal variations in the shape of the choroid plexus should not be misinterpreted as hemorrhage.[24] Rarely, hemorrhage within the choroid plexus may cause globular regions of hypo- (cystlike) or hyperechogenicity[7]; however, small isolated choroid plexus hemorrhages have no particular clinical significance. Doppler interrogation may also help to differentiate hypervascular choroid plexus from hypovascular clot.[24]

Choroid Plexus Cysts

Choroid plexus cysts occur as isolated normal variants in about 1% of pregnancies.[14,25] In an otherwise healthy infant with no other structural

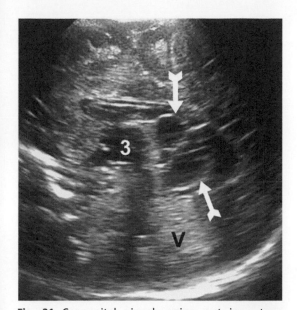

Fig. 21. Congenital pineal region cyst in a term newborn with history of hydrocephalus on fetal ultrasound. Sagittal ultrasound image identifies a multilocular cystic lesion in the pineal region (*arrows*). Magnetic resonance image (not shown) confirmed a congenital midline cyst associated with extensive cortical dysplasia and heterotopic gray matter. The cerebellar vermis (V) and third ventricle (3) are indicated.

abnormalities, they are of no clinical significance.[14,25] Choroid plexus cysts are typically round, measure less than 1 cm, and vary in number (**Fig. 26**).[14,26] Larger (>1 cm), multiple, and bilateral cysts are more likely associated with a chromosomal aneuploidy, such as trisomy 18.[3]

Periventricular Connatal and Subependymal Cysts

The terminology in the literature describing periventricular cysts has been applied inconsistently. In this section, we review this terminology and discuss the most common types of periventricular cysts. Periventricular cystic lesions include connatal cysts (a normal variant); pathologic lesions, such as subependymal cysts; and periventricular leukomalacia (**Fig. 27**).[14] Connatal cysts have also been called subfrontal or frontal horn cysts and have been categorized as subependymal cysts by some investigators. For the purposes of this manuscript, we will refer to connatal cysts separately from subependymal cysts because they differ in pathologic origin and location.

The formation of connatal cysts, which are located adjacent to the superolateral margins of the frontal horns of the lateral ventricles, is believed due to approximation or coarctation of the walls of the frontal horns of the lateral ventricles just proximal to the external angles.[14,27,28] The cysts are most likely a normal,

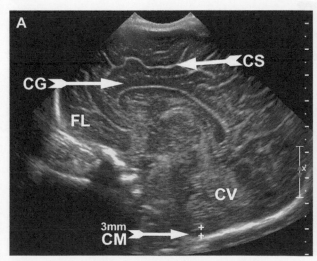
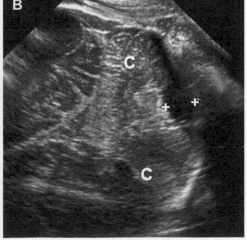

Fig. 22. Cisterna magna in a 2-day-old term infant. (*A*) Sagittal ultrasound demonstrates the normal cisterna magna (CM and *calipers*) just inferior to the cerebellar vermis (CV). Also noted are the cingulate sulcus (CS), cingulate gyrus (CG), and frontal lobe (FL). (*B*) Posterior fontanelle axial ultrasound confirms the normal anatomy with increased eloquence, including the cerebellar hemispheres (C) and normal cisterna magna (*calipers*).

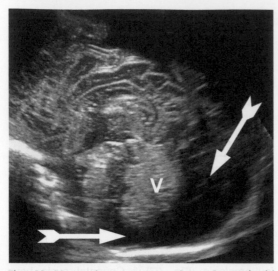

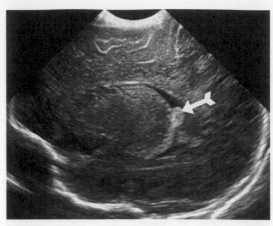

Fig. 25. Lobulated choroid plexus in a term infant. Parasagittal image of the lateral ventricle demonstrates the normal choroid plexus, which has a "lumpy" contour (*arrow*).

Fig. 23. Mega cisterna magna in a 3-month-old infant. Sagittal ultrasound demonstrates a hypoechoic fluid collection (*arrows*) posterior to the normal cerebellar vermis (V).

ependyma-lined neurodevelopmental variant.[29,30] They are usually seen in the first few days of life and may undergo a period of enlargement followed by spontaneous resolution.[28,30] Furthermore, when seen in isolation, they are of no proven clinical significance.[29] Key imaging features include bilateral, symmetric, multiple cysts, often lined up like a string of pearls along the margin of the frontal horn anterior to the foramina of Monro (**Fig. 28**).[14]

Cysts located at the caudothalamic groove and posterior to foramen of Monro are likely to represent a subependymal cyst (**Fig. 29**).[14] Subependymal cysts can be classified as congenital (germinolytic) or acquired (posthemorrhagic). Unfortunately, without a documented history of prior grade I germinal matrix hemorrhage, the two types of subependymal cysts cannot be distinguished with imaging.[2,14] Posthemorrhagic cysts occur at the caudothalamic groove and measure 2 to 11 mm.[2] The cause of congenital subependymal, or germinolytic, cysts is not known, but investigators have suggested that the

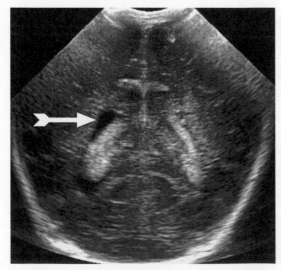

Fig. 24. Asymmetric ventricle size in a premature infant born at 34 weeks gestational age. Coronal ultrasound shows that the right lateral ventricle (*arrow*) is slightly larger than the left, although both are normal in size, measuring less than 10 mm.

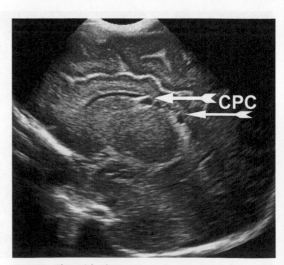

Fig. 26. Choroid plexus cysts in a term infant with history of two-vessel cord and hypoplastic left heart. Parasagittal image of the lateral ventricle identifies multiple well-defined anechoic cysts within the choroid plexus (CPC).

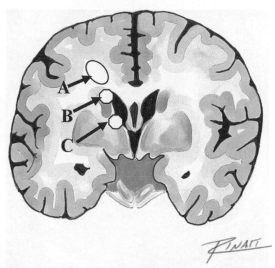

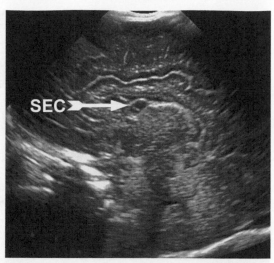

Fig. 27. Schematic drawing demonstrating the expected various locations of periventricular leukomalacia (A), connatal cyst (B), and subependymal cyst (C). (*Courtesy of* Reza Zintai, MD.)

Fig. 29. Subependymal cyst in a term newborn. Sagittal ultrasound image reveals a round, well-defined anechoic subependymal cyst (SEC) at the caudothalamic groove.

Hyperechoic White Matter Pseudolesions

cysts result from prior in utero hypoxic, hemorrhagic, or infectious insult, such as cytomegalovirus and rubella.[14,31] Germinolytic subependymal cysts have also been associated with genetic disorders; metabolic diseases, such as Zellweger syndrome; and maternal cocaine intake. The cysts have been reported in isolation in healthy newborns as well.[2,14,31] If the cysts are located within the deep white matter above the lateral ventricles, periventricular leukomalacia should be the predominant consideration.[14]

Hyperechoic white matter pseudolesions may occur along the edge of a gyrus secondary to imaging a sulcus tangentially.[3] The pitfall of hyperechoic white matter pseudolesions can be avoided by rotating the transducer 90° to the hyperechoic region, which will confirm a normal-appearing gyrus on the orthogonal view (**Fig. 30**).[3] In general, lesions identified on head ultrasound must be seen in two planes to be confirmed as truly abnormal, rather than artifact.

Prominent Periventricular Halo

The normal prominent hyperechoic periventricular white matter, or periventricular halo, runs parallel to the lateral ventricles (**Fig. 31**). To avoid misinterpreting the periventricular halo as abnormal, the clinician must compare echogenicity to the adjacent choroid plexus. In the past, the normal periventricular halo was distinguished from pathology by echogenicity less than the adjacent choroid plexus.[3,8] However, with modern ultrasound equipment, image quality has improved to such a degree that borderline changes in the periventricular halo, such as asymmetric, heterogenous, or globular subtle abnormal echogenicity, may be identified. A linear, high-resolution transducer may help distinguish between the normal and abnormal periventricular halo. When pathology is present, it is most often due to periventricular hemorrhage, periventricular leukomalacia, or both.[3,32]

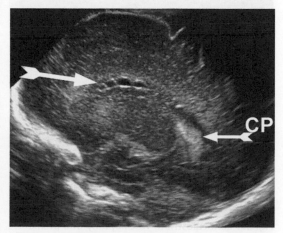

Fig. 28. Connatal cysts in a preterm infant. Parasagittal image shows four anechoic connatal cysts lined up in a typical string-of-pearls configuration along the floor of the frontal horn of left lateral ventricle (*large arrow*). Small arrow indicates the choroid plexus (CP).

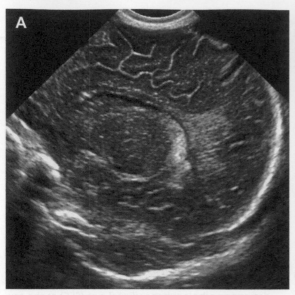
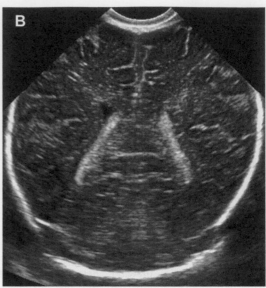

Fig. 30. Hyperechoic white matter pseudolesion in a 2-day-old term infant. (*A*) Sagittal image demonstrates a region of increased echogenicity adjacent to the posterior aspect of the lateral ventricle, which is absent on the orthogonal coronal image (*B*). Also of note is the excellent visualization of the three echogenic layers of the brain, already described in Figure 2, including the thin linear pia, which overlies the cortical gray matter and the slightly deeper, more hyperechoic white matter.

Lenticulostriate Vasculopathy

Lenticulostriate vasculopathy, occasionally seen on ultrasound, is often a nonspecific, isolated, incidental finding. It may be unilateral or bilateral, and is seen as branching, linear, or punctate areas of echogenicity (**Fig. 32**).[33–35] Pathologically

lenticulostriate vasculopathy represents thickened walls of the medium-sized lenticulostriate arteries with deposition of amorphous basophilic material, iron, and calcium, and vessel damage.[33–35] Lenticulostriate vasculopathy is a nonspecific finding without a known specific cause. It has been described in association with

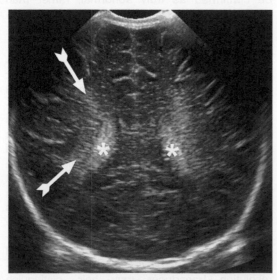

Fig. 31. Periventricular halo in a term infant. Coronal ultrasound image reveals increased echogenicity within the periventricular white matter (*arrows*) running parallel to the margins of the lateral ventricles. Also noted is the choroid plexus (*asterisks*).

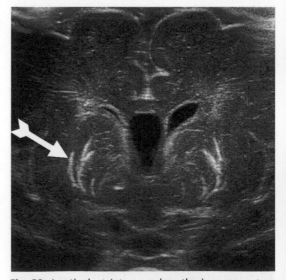

Fig. 32. Lenticulostriate vasculopathy in a premature infant born at 33 weeks gestational age. Coronal ultrasound image obtained with a linear transducer shows extensive bilateral, branching, linear echogenicity within the thalami (*arrow*). The cavum septum pellucidum is noted between the frontal horns.

underlying conditions, such as fetal TORCH infections (toxoplasmosis, rubella, cytomegalovirus, herpes simplex, and syphilis), chromosome abnormalities, malformations, and hypoxic ischemic states, though no one has yet proven that any of these underlying conditions cause lenticulostriate vasculopathy. Lenticulostriate vasculopathy is often seen as an isolated abnormality of unknown etiology.[35] While the short-term outcome of infants with isolated lenticulostriate vasculopathy is good, there may be associated long-term sequelae, such as attention-deficit/hyperactivity disorders and tics.[35]

REFERENCES

1. Shuman WP, Rogers JV, Mack LA, et al. Real-time sonographic sector scanning of the neonatal cranium: technique and normal anatomy. AJR Am J Roentgenol 1981;137:821.

2. Daneman A, Epelman M, Blaser S, et al. Imaging of the brain in full-term neonates: Does sonography still play a role? Pediatr Radiol 2006;36:636.

3. Segal M. Pediatric sonography. 53rd edition. Philadelphia: Lippencott Williams and Wilkins; 2002.

4. Rumack C, Wilson S, Charboneau J, et al, editors. Diagnostic ultrasound, vol. 2. 3rd edition. St. Louis (MO): Mosby; 2005. p.1623–702.

5. Lowe LH, Bulas DI. Transcranial Doppler imaging in children: sickle cell screening and beyond. Pediatr Radiol 2005;35:54.

6. Huang BY, Castillo M. Hypoxic-ischemic brain injury: imaging findings from birth to adulthood. Radiographics 2008;28:417.

7. Slovis TL, Kuhns LR. Real-time sonography of the brain through the anterior fontanelle. AJR Am J Roentgenol 1981;136:277.

8. Grant EG, Schellinger D, Richardson JD, et al. Echogenic periventricular halo: normal sonographic finding or neonatal cerebral hemorrhage. AJR Am J Roentgenol 1983;140:793.

9. Grant EG, Schellinger D, Borts FT, et al. Real-time sonography of the neonatal and infant head. AJR Am J Roentgenol 1981;136:265.

10. Bulas DI, Vezina GL. Preterm anoxic injury. Radiologic evaluation. Radiol Clin North Am 1999;37:1147.

11. Soetaert AM, Lowe LH, Formen C. Pediatric cranial Doppler sonography in children: non-sickle cell applications. Curr Probl Diagn Radiol 2009;38:218.

12. Allison JW, Faddis LA, Kinder DL, et al. Intracranial resistive index (RI) values in normal term infants during the first day of life. Pediatr Radiol 2000;30:618.

13. Yazici B, Erdogmus B, Tugay A. Cerebral blood flow measurements of the extracranial carotid and vertebral arteries with doppler ultrasonography in healthy adults. Diagn Interv Radiol 2005;11:195.

14. Epelman M, Daneman A, Blaser SI, et al. Differential diagnosis of intracranial cystic lesions at head US: correlation with CT and MR imaging. Radiographics 2006;26:173.

15. Bronshtein M, Weiner Z. Prenatal diagnosis of dilated cava septi pellucidi et vergae: associated anomalies, differential diagnosis, and pregnancy outcome. Obstet Gynecol 1992;80:838.

16. Chen CY, Chen FH, Lee CC, et al. Sonographic characteristics of the cavum velum interpositum. AJNR Am J Neuroradiol 1998;19:1631.

17. Osborn A. Handbook of neuroradiology. St. Louis (MO): Mosby- Year Book; 1991.

18. Goodwin L, Quisling RG. The neonatal cisterna magna: ultrasonic evaluation. Radiology 1983;149:691.

19. Bernard JP, Moscoso G, Renier D, et al. Cystic malformations of the posterior fossa. Prenat Diagn 2001;21:1064.

20. Middleton WD, Kurtz AB, Hertzbert BS. Ultrasound: the requisites. 2nd edition. St. Louis (MO): Mosby-Year book; 2009. p. 377.

21. Winchester P, Brill PW, Cooper R, et al. Prevalence of "compressed" and asymmetric lateral ventricles in healthy full-term neonates: sonographic study. AJR Am J Roentgenol 1986;146:471.

22. Horbar JD, Leahy KA, Lucey JF. Ultrasound identification of lateral ventricular asymmetry in the human neonate. J Clin Ultrasound 1983;11:67.

23. Koeda T, Ando Y, Takashima S, et al. Changes in the lateral ventricle with the head position: ultrasonographic observation. Neuroradiology 1988;30:315.

24. Di Salvo DN. A new view of the neonatal brain: clinical utility of supplemental neurologic US imaging windows. Radiographics 2001;21:943.

25. Ostlere SJ, Irving HC, Lilford RJ. Fetal choroid plexus cysts: a report of 100 cases. Radiology 1990;175:753.

26. van Baalen A, Versmold H. Choroid plexus cyst: comparison of new ultrasound technique with old histological finding. Arch Dis Child 2004;89:426.

27. Enriquez G, Correa F, Lucaya J, et al. Potential pitfalls in cranial sonography. Pediatr Radiol 2003;33:110.

28. Rosenfeld DL, Schonfeld SM, Underberg-Davis S. Coarctation of the lateral ventricles: an alternative explanation for subependymal pseudocysts. Pediatr Radiol 1997;27:895.

29. Pal BR, Preston PR, Morgan ME, et al. Frontal horn thin walled cysts in preterm neonates are benign. Arch Dis Child Fetal Neonatal Ed 2001;85:F187.

30. Chang CL, Chiu NC, Ho CS, et al. Frontal horn cysts in normal neonates. Brain Dev 2006;28:426.

31. Makhoul IR, Zmora O, Tamir A, et al. Congenital subependymal pseudocysts: own data and meta-analysis of the literature. Isr Med Assoc J 2001; 3:178.

32. DiPietro MA, Brody BA, Teele RL. Peritrigonal echogenic "blush" on cranial sonography: pathologic correlates. AJR Am J Roentgenol 1986;146:1067.

33. Cabanas F, Pellicer A, Morales C, et al. New pattern of hyperechogenicity in thalamus and basal ganglia studied by color doppler flow imaging. Pediatr Neurol 1994;10:109.

34. Coley BD, Rusin JA, Boue DR. Importance of hypoxic/ischemic conditions in the development of cerebral lenticulostriate vasculopathy. Pediatr Radiol 2000;30:846.

35. Makhoul IR, Eisenstein I, Sujov P, et al. Neonatal lenticulostriate vasculopathy: further characterisation. Arch Dis Child Fetal Neonatal Ed 2003;88:F410.

Neurosonography

Lori L. Barr, MD[a,b,*]

KEYWORDS

• Neurosonogram • Neurosonography • Head ultrasound

Neurosonography remains the preferred method of early imaging of the brain while the fontanelles remain open because of low cost, portability, and safety. This article provides a framework for expansion of the ability to detect the gamut of neuropathology affecting infants. This skill is best mastered by actual scanning of patients after initial screening by a highly proficient sonographer. In all conditions—congenital, infectious, neoplastic, and injury—neurosonography is often the first step. Additional cross-sectional imaging modalities are used to evaluate structures and functions not easily imaged with neurosonography, such as the subarachnoid space for hemorrhage; preoperative planning evaluation for tumors or space-occupying lesions; or where demyelination is questioned.

Advances in neurosonography, such as 3-dimensional (3D) imaging,[1] quantitative tissue characterization,[2] and contrast use,[3,4] are still in the investigative phase of clinical implementation. Continued research in these specialty areas will more accurately measure meaningful parameters with regard to patient outcome.

CONGENITAL ANOMALIES

The division of congenital malformations into 4 subgroups based on embryologic neurologic development timing as proposed by Van der Knapp and Valk[5] remains the accepted standard for division of congenital malformations into categories. The 4 subgroups are: dorsal induction (primary neurulation 3–4 weeks gestational age [GA]; secondary neurulation, 4–40 weeks GA); ventral induction (5–8 weeks GA); neuronal proliferation, differentiation, and histogenesis (8–16 weeks GA); and neuronal migration (8–20 weeks

GA through 1 year after birth). Discussed here are anomalies where ultrasound is helpful in patient evaluation.

Dorsal Induction

Closure defects

Pre- and postnatal imaging are important because of the fragile coverings over the otherwise exposed central nervous system (CNS) in patients with cephalocele, meningocele, myelomeningocele, and other closure defects (**Fig. 1**). Prenatal scanning of fetuses between weeks 11 and 13 GA should allow visualization of the fourth ventricle as a measurable intracranial translucency in the mid-sagittal view that is now popular for measurement of the nuchal translucency. If the fourth ventricle is not visible, this indicates a neural tube defect.[6] Magnetic resonance (MR) imaging is the modality of choice after birth. Two goals of imaging of the actual cephalocele, meningocele, or myelomeningocele are to identify the extent of the neural tube defect and the contents of the sac. Specifically, the question is whether there are neural elements included in the sac as surgical repair is altered.

Chiari malformations

Neurosonography is useful in identification, surgical intervention, and follow-up of Chiari malformations. Infants with Chiari I may be asymptomatic with the finding discovered incidentally (**Fig. 2**). If these patients become symptomatic, intraoperative neurosonography can be instrumental in assessment. The surgeon wants to know how far down into the cervical canal the tonsils herniate with cerebrospinal fluid (CSF) pulsation to minimize the development of a syrinx. Infants with Chiari II, dysgenesis of the hindbrain,

[a] Department of Radiology, The University of Texas Medical Branch, 301 University Boulevard, Galveston, TX 77555, USA
[b] Austin Radiology Association, 10900 Stonelake Boulevard, Suite 250, Austin, TX 78759, USA
* Austin Radiology Association, 10900 Stonelake Boulevard, Suite 250, Austin, TX 78759.
E-mail address: barrlmd@ausrad.com

Ultrasound Clin 4 (2009) 513–532
doi:10.1016/j.cult.2009.11.006
1556-858X/09/$ – see front matter © 2009 Elsevier Inc. All rights reserved.

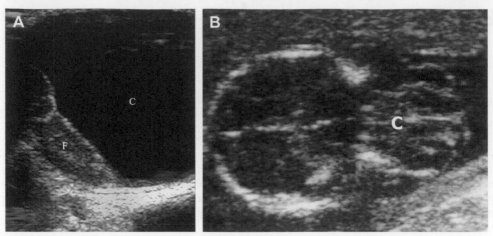

Fig. 1. Cephalocele. (A) Left frontal sagittal neurosonogram in a newborn with large soft scalp mass at birth demonstrates an encephalocele with both cerebrospinal fluid (C) and a portion of the frontal lobe (F). (B) Coronal transabdominal fetal neurosonogram through the posterior aspect of the head demonstrates a large occipital encephalocele containing most of the cerebellum (C). Note the lack of echogenic calvarium around the cerebellum.

are usually studied at birth in conjunction with spina bifida. Neurosonography is useful for diagnosis of secondary hydrocephalus over time after closure of the neural tube defect. Sonographic findings in Chiari II include downward displacement and enlargement of the fourth ventricle, prominent massa intermedia, obliteration of cisterna magna, inferior pointing of the anterior horns of the lateral ventricles, and interdigitation of the falx cerebri (**Fig. 3**). Other commonly associated findings are colpocephaly, hydrocephalus,

corpus callosum dysgenesis, and syringohydromyelia. Serial neurosonograms are performed with the same image depth so that the size of the ventricles is easily compared, unless 3D imaging is used. Hydrocephalus in these cases is usually caused by aqueductal stenosis (**Fig. 4**).

Ventral Induction

Ventral induction leads to formation of the hindbrain, midbrain, forebrain, and face. Abnormalities of ventral induction include abnormalities of the hypothalamic-pituitary axis, cerebellar malformations, dorsal cysts, holoprosencephaly, and pellucidal agenesis/dysgenesis. Abnormalities of the hypothalamic-pituitary axis are very difficult to see with ultrasound while the other entities are only detectable on neurosonograms if the operator is familiar with the possible diagnosis and associated findings. When neurosonography is performed with this knowledge, MR imaging may be postponed until later in infancy, when it is of more value to the patient's clinical care to assess the progress of myelination at the same time.

Cerebellar anomalies
Cerebellar anomalies are disorders of ventral induction. Prenatal 3D ultrasound is very promising in accurate diagnosis of these abnormalities.[1] Cystic posterior fossa malformations are a result of dysgenesis of the paleocerebellum (flocculi and vermis), and are common. These malformations include the Dandy-Walker spectrum and mega cisterna magna. Isolated vermian anomalies and Joubert syndrome are also paleocerebellar in

Fig. 2. Chiari I malformation. Sagittal neurosonogram demonstrates absence of fluid in cisterna magna (arrow). Note that the fourth ventricle is caudally displaced and somewhat flattened (curved arrow).

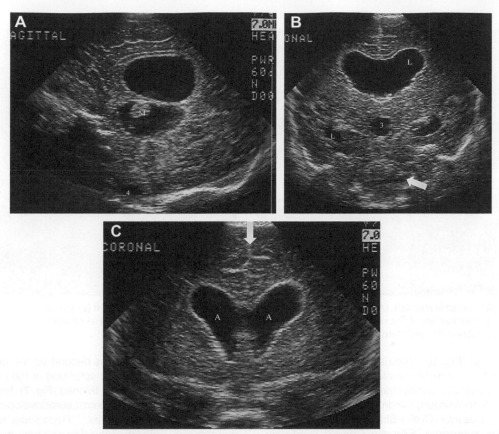

Fig. 3. Chiari II malformation. (*A*) Sagittal neurosonogram of a neonate demonstrates downward displacement and enlargement of the fourth ventricle (**4**) and prominence of massa intermedia (M). Cisterna magna is obliterated. (*B*) Posterior coronal image through the cerebrum and the cerebellum demonstrates prominence of the lateral (L) and the third (**3**) ventricles with an abnormally shaped fourth ventricle (*arrow*). (*C*) Anterior coronal image through the infant's head demonstrates inferior pointing of the anterior horns (A) of the lateral ventricles and interdigitation of the falx cerebri (*arrow*).

origin. The neocerebellum is composed of the remainder of the cerebellar hemispheres. Dysgenesis of the neocerebellum results in combined cerebellovermian hypoplasia, cerebellar hemispheric aplasia/hypoplasia, and cerebellar dysplasia.

Dandy-Walker spectrum The Dandy-Walker spectrum includes Dandy-Walker malformation, Dandy-Walker variant, and mega cisterna magna. The most severe form, Dandy-Walker malformation, consists of cystic dilatation of the fourth ventricle, upward displacement of the tentorium resulting in an enlarged posterior fossa, and vermian agenesis (**Fig. 5**). These findings are usually complicated by hydrocephalus over time. Cerebral anomalies are associated in 68% of cases.[7] Variant describes cases that do not demonstrate the classic Dandy-Walker malformation findings. Mega cisterna magna is enlargement of the cisterna magna without associated anomalies, and is considered a normal variant with a good

long-term outcome. Outcome is very poor with Dandy-Walker syndrome and Variant, mainly due to associated anomalies.[8]

Cerebellar and vermian hypoplasia and dysplasia A new classification of cerebellar anomalies was proposed by Patel and Barkovich in 2003.[9] Recognition of hypoplasia versus dysplasia and diffuse versus focal disease is important in separating infants with associated cerebral anomalies from those with isolated cerebellar anomalies. The presence of associated anomalies is linked to poor prognosis. Postnatal MR imaging is the gold standard for the classification, and differentiation of hypoplasia from dysplasia is not reliable by ultrasound. Agenesis is recognized by the absence of the echogenic vermis and cerebellar hemispheres. Hypoplasia of the vermis is characterized by flattening of the inferior vermis on the midline sagittal view. Asymmetry of the cerebellar hemispheres or small size is a clue for cerebellar

A

B

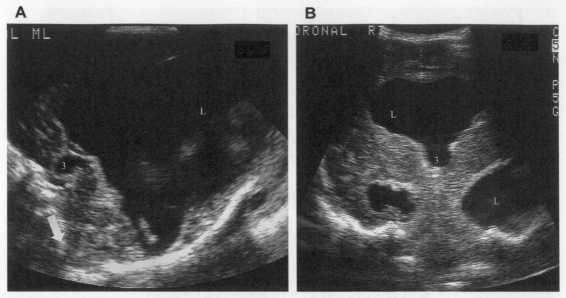

Fig. 4. Aqueductal stenosis. (*A*) Sagittal neurosonogram shows enlargement of the third (**3**) and lateral (**L**) ventricles. Note herniation of the cerebellar tonsils into foramen magnum (*arrow*). (*B*) Coronal neurosonogram shows enlarged lateral (**L**) and third (**3**) ventricles.

hypoplasia (**Fig. 6**). Three syndromes are associated with complete vermian agenesis: cerebro-ocular muscular syndromes, Joubert syndrome, and Walker-Warburg syndrome. Vermian agenesis may be present in Coffin-Siris syndrome, cryptophthalmos syndrome, Ellis-van Creveld syndrome, and Meckel-Gruber syndrome.[10]

Corpus callosum aplasia/hypoplasia
This disorder of ventral induction is the result of impaired cleavage of the prosencephalon. Aplasia is associated with seizures and mental retardation.

Neurosonographic findings depend on the portion (rostrum, genu, body, and splenium) of the corpus callosum that is absent or thinned (**Fig. 7**). Isolated agenesis has a good long-term neurodevelopmental prognosis in 80% of cases.[11] Hypoplasia is also common and both are associated with preterm birth, intrauterine infection, and advanced maternal age.[12]

Holoprosencephaly
Holoprosencephaly is a disorder of ventral induction with incomplete cleavage of the prosencephalon. There is a high association of midline defects

A

B

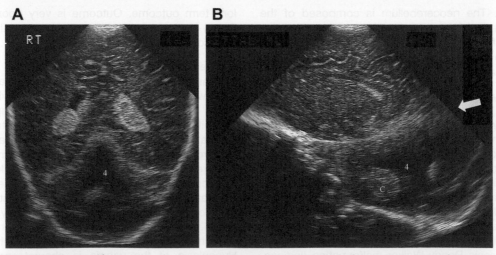

Fig. 5. Dandy-Walker malformation. (*A*) Posterior coronal neurosonogram demonstrates an enlarged posterior fossa and cystic dilation of the fourth ventricle (**4**). Cerebellar vermis is absent. (*B*) Right parasagittal neurosonogram shows the uplifted tentorium (*arrow*), large fourth ventricle (**4**), and a portion of the right cerebellar hemisphere (**C**). Cerebellar vermis is more echogenic than the hemispheres.

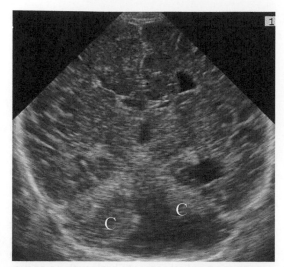

Fig. 6. Cerebellovermian hypoplasia. Coronal neuro-sonogram demonstrates small asymmetric cerebellar hemispheres (C) and absence of the vermis. This patient also has findings of Dandy-Walker malformation and absent corpus callosum.

involving face and body, with environmental factors and 7 genes implicated as causes. Prenatal diagnosis rests on ultrasound and MR imaging.[13] Many parents opt for pregnancy termination. Postnatal neurosonography and MR imaging help the multidisciplinary team manage the patient's related difficulties.[14]

The most severe form is alobar holoprosencephaly. The brain consists of only a flat mass of anteriorly fused cerebral hemispheres in the frontal region and a monoventricle that communicates with a large dorsal cyst. The falx cerebri is absent and the thalami are fused. Convolutional markings are sparse with a smooth appearance to the brain surface. There are often associated migrational anomalies. Vascular abnormalities include absent or single internal cerebral arteries, absence of the cerebral vein, superior sinus, sagittal sinus, and the straight sinus. This form of holoprosencephaly is associated with trisomy 13 and with trisomy 18.

A less severe form is semilobar holoprosencephaly where the interhemispheric fissure is developed posteriorly but incomplete anteriorly. Partial fusion of the thalami along the floor of the malformed third ventricle is a hallmark finding (**Fig. 8**). A single ventricle is present. Portions of the septum pellucidum and corpus callosum may or may not be present.

The mildest form of holoprosencephaly is lobar. The anteroinferior portion of the interhemispheric fissure is incomplete, and there is interdigitation of the falx cerebri. The cerebral cortex is fused at the frontal pole with an absent septum pellucidum. The corpus callosum is usually malformed. Associated migrational anomalies such as gray matter heterotopias are more easily evaluated with high-frequency transducers in the 10- to 13-MHz frequency range.

Pellucidal agenesis and dysgenesis

Although primary agenesis of the septum pellucidum does occur, secondary destruction is more common. This destruction may happen after trauma, inflammation, or ventricular obstruction. The coronal view is the most useful in demonstrating the absence of the septum pellucidum (**Fig. 9**). Many anomalies are associated with absence of the septum pellucidum, including aqueductal stenosis with secondary hydrocephalus, callosal agenesis, Chiari II, migrational

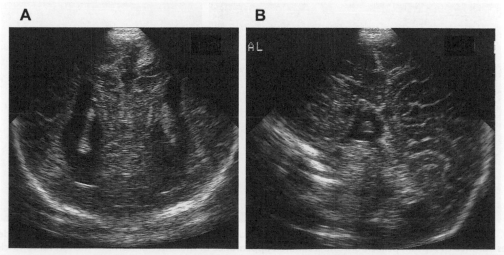

A   B

Fig. 7. Corpus callosum aplasia. (*A*) Coronal neurosonogram shows a parallel orientation of the lateral ventricles. (*B*) Sagittal view demonstrates a radial array of the sulci and absence of corpus callosum.

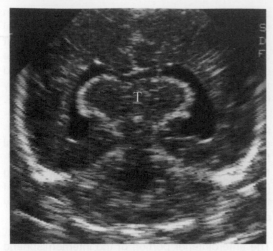

Fig. 8. Semilobar holoprosencephaly. Coronal neuro-sonogram demonstrates fusion of the thalami (T) and a monoventricle.

anomalies, and septo-optic dysplasia. Septo-optic dysplasia associates the absent septum pellucidum with hypoplasia of the optic canals, chiasm, and nerves. Most individuals with septo-optic dysplasia also have hypothalamic/pituitary disorders.[15]

Migration Anomalies

Between the third and fifth months of life, disorders of neuronal migration occur when the neurons fail to migrate to their final locations within the cerebral cortex. Many of these anomalies represent genetic malformations, and are associated with syndromes.[16] Most present with epilepsy, hypotonia, or developmental delay.[17,18]

Heterotopias
When there is an arrest in the normal radial migration of neurons and glial tissue from the periventricular germinal matrix to the cortex, heterotopic gray matter occurs. These arrests are only detected with high-frequency transducers and a high index of suspicion, as they appear so similar to the normal gray matter. Heterotopias may be bandlike or nodular (**Fig. 10**), and range in location from subpial to subependymal regions.

Lissencephaly
Lissencephaly is a severe migrational anomaly that results in seizures in all infants, and death before the age of 2 years for most infants. Agyria describes an entirely smooth brain with no convolutional markings (**Fig. 11**). Pachygyria results in a few flat gyri. The normal prenatal brain is very smooth at 25 weeks' GA; thus, accurate estimation of the preterm infant gestational age is essential in making an accurate neurosonographic diagnosis of lissencephaly.

Polymicrogyria
Cortical dysplasia with a "cobblestoned" appearance is referred to as polymicrogyria. Clinical symptoms vary with lesion location. The cortex appears slightly thickened and is similar to pachygyria (**Fig. 12**). One should look for large draining veins caused by a persistent fetal vascular pattern in the leptomeninges covering the abnormal cortex. Identification of this finding should prompt MR evaluation.

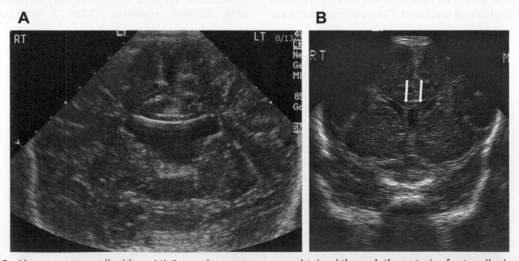

Fig. 9. Absent septum pellucidum. (*A*) Coronal neurosonogram obtained through the anterior fontanelle demonstrates absence of septum pellucidum and a squared appearance of the anterior horns of the lateral ventricles. (*B*) Coronal neurosonogram demonstrating the normal septi pellucidi (*arrows*) separated by cavum septum pellucidum for comparison.

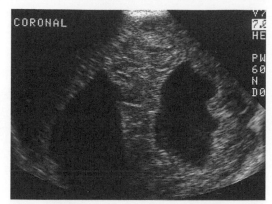

Fig. 10. Gray matter heterotopia. Coronal neurosonogram demonstrates nodular foci of gray matter studding the wall of the left lateral ventricle.

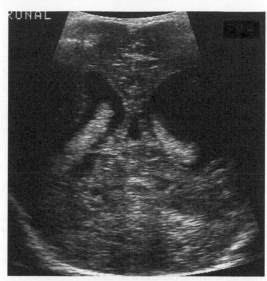

Fig. 12. Cortical dysplasia. Coronal neurosonogram demonstrates areas of irregular gyri and some featureless areas without the uniformity seen in lissencephaly. Pachygyria looks the same.

Schizencephaly

Schizencephaly is a brain cleft lined by gray matter. Defects may be large with associated developmental delay, or small with mild spasticity or hypotonia.[19] Lesions are divided into separated lips or fused clefts. The fused clefts are referred to as type 1 or closed-lip schizencephaly and the open lips are referred to as type II (**Fig. 13**). Associations include mineralizing vasculopathy, absence of the septum pellucidum, cortical dysplasia, and gray matter heterotopias. This lesion is associated with cytomegalovirus infection.

Neuronal Proliferation and Differentiation

Aqueductal stenosis, the phakomatoses, congenital vascular malformations, and congenital tumors arise during this period of increase in cell number and cell type.

Aqueductal stenosis

Primary aqueductal stenosis occurs from abnormalities in the neuronal differentiation or proliferation of the periaqueductal gray matter but is more commonly caused by scarring after compression, hemorrhage, or infection. Whether imaging is

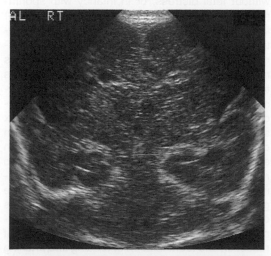

Fig. 11. Lissencephaly. Coronal neurosonogram demonstrates a featureless cortex without sulcation.

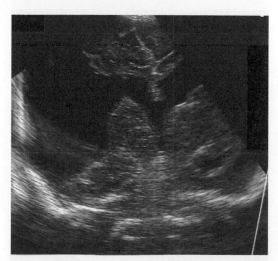

Fig. 13. Schizencephaly. Coronal neurosonogram shows a Type II open lip schizencephaly of the right frontotemporal region. Note free communication of the right lateral ventricle with the extra-axial fluid.

performed prenatally or postnatally, the asymmetric enlargement of the lateral and third ventricles with a normal-sized fourth ventricle is the hallmark pattern (see **Fig. 4**). Differentiation from holoprosencephaly may be assisted by use of the mastoid view (**Fig. 14**).[20] For assessment over time, it is important to keep the transfontanelle image depth constant between serial scans for easy comparison unless 3D ultrasound is employed.

Phakomatoses

The phakomatoses describe syndromes with abnormal proliferation of ectodermal, mesodermal, and neuroectodermal components that affect the brain globally and that lead to the development of small tumors within the CNS, genitourinary system, and the skin. Examples are Sturge-Weber syndrome and tuberous sclerosis.

Sturge-Weber syndrome Patients have a facial port-wine nevus associated with an ipsilateral leptomeningeal angioma and seizures in the first year of life. Sturge-Weber syndrome is also called encephalotrigeminal angiomatosis. The affected hemisphere demonstrates decreased cortical volume, enlarged choroid plexus, and serpiginous echo densities in the brain periphery (**Fig. 15**). The earliest ultrasound finding may be unilateral periventricular increased echogenicity.[21]

Tuberous sclerosis Tuberous sclerosis is a multisystem inherited disorder with multiple tumorlike lesions in the brain, eyes, heart, kidneys, lungs, and skin. Pre- and postnatal sonography is instrumental in low-cost follow-up of these masses, because

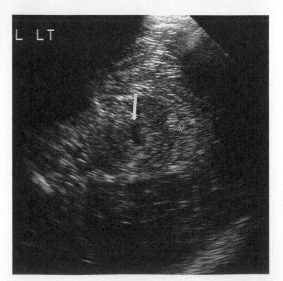

Fig. 14. Mastoid view. Axial view of the normal fourth ventricle (*arrow*) from a left mastoid approach. Note the echogenic cerebellar vermis (V).

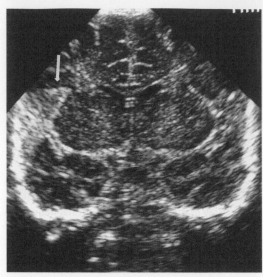

Fig. 15. Sturge-Weber Syndrome. Coronal neurosonogram demonstrates asymmetry of the sylvian fissures and a wedge-shaped area of increased echogenicity on the right. This is the leptomeningeal angioma (*arrow*).

many have the potential to develop into more aggressive lesions like subependymal giant cell astrocytoma and renal cell carcinoma.[22] Neurosonograms are often obtained when an infant presents with nonspecific neurologic symptoms. Findings include periventricular subependymal nodules (usually calcified) near the foramen of Munro and cortical hamartomas, both of which appear iso- to hyperechoic with respect to normal brain (**Fig. 16**).[23]

Vascular malformations

Vascular malformations may present in utero as dural sinus enlargement or thrombosis with or without fetal distress, or in infancy with spontaneous intracranial hemorrhage or congestive heart failure. Included are brain arteriovenous malformations, cavernous malformations, dural arteriovenous fistulas, Galenic malformations, venous malformations, and venous varices.[24] Limitations to identification depend on location of the malformation, neurosonographic equipment, and protocols used. Transcranial color-coded duplex sonography has an overall sensitivity of 78% in one study but is not sensitive enough to be an effective screening tool.[25] Although magnetic resonance and computed tomographic arteriography are showing the potential to replace it, the gold standard for preoperative planning remains conventional angiography. Intraoperative sonography is important in assessing completeness of resection and identification of feeding and draining vessels. Sensitivity has increased with 3D sonoangiography.[26] Focal areas of increased or

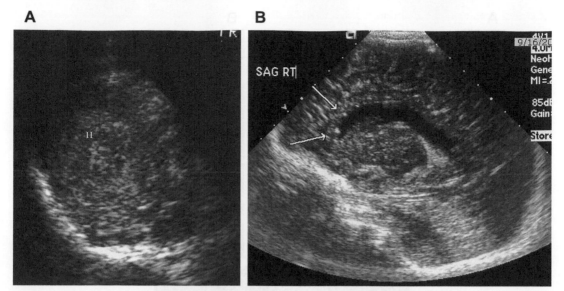

Fig. 16. Tuberous sclerosis. (*A*) Coronal neurosonogram of a neonate obtained intraoperatively demonstrates the similarity of the echogenicity of the hamartoma (H) to normal brain. (*B*) Parasagittal neurosonogram in a different toddler with seizures demonstrates subependymal tubers (*arrows*).

decreased echogenicity appear on gray-scale images with obvious focal increased vascularity on color or power Doppler (**Fig. 17**).

INFECTION

Diagnosis of pre- and postnatal CNS infection is almost always made clinically. Common infections during the prenatal period include those described in the TORCH complex (toxoplasmosis, rubella, cytomegalovirus [CMV], herpes simplex, with the "O" including hepatitis B, HIV, Parvovirus B19, syphilis, and varicella-zoster). Perinatal infections are commonly caused by *Escherichia coli*, group B streptococcus, and *Listeria monocytogenes*; all are causes of neonatal meningitis. Ultrasound findings are similar between these entities, and may suggest an infectious etiology in clinically silent cases. Otherwise the role of imaging is to reveal complications of infection. Complications include abscess, calcifications, cerebritis, encephalomalacia, hydrocephalus, infarctions, ischemia, malformation, mineralizing vasculopathy, and septations within the ventricles. Some of these complications have prognostic implications. In preterm infants, the association of intrauterine infection and periventricular hemorrhagic infarction is associated with mortality, regardless of optimal treatment.[27]

Intrauterine Infection

Cytomegalovirus
This is the most prevalent cause of intrauterine infection worldwide, and humans are the only

carriers found to date. This member of the Herpes virus family spreads through body fluids, including breast milk. Birth prevalence is estimated at 0.7%, and 12.7% of infected newborns develop clinical signs of infection. Permanent sequelae occur in 40% to 58% of symptomatic patients and in 13.5% of asymptomatic patients.[28] In the CNS the target of the virus is the germinal matrix, because its modus operandi is to affect undifferentiated cells during migration, proliferation, and differentiation. The hallmark of infection is the presence of calcifications that may be in the basal ganglia, cortex, periventricular subependymal location, and subcortical.[29] Bilateral periventricular calcifications surrounded by hypoechoic rings are characteristic of CMV infection (**Fig. 18**). Another common finding in CMV infection is mineralizing vasculopathy, where microscopic mineral deposits occur along the lenticulostriate vessels in the basil ganglia, causing a candelabra appearance of echogenic lines (**Fig. 19**). These lines are not specific for CMV infection and also occur with asphyxia, cyanotic heart disease, Down syndrome, fetal alcohol syndrome, ischemia, nonimmune hydrops, and trisomy 13. CMV infection is also associated with anomalies of migration and neuronal proliferation/differentiation.

Toxoplasma gondii
Toxoplasmosis is caused by invasion of the protozoan *Toxoplasma gondii* into the human system, usually by exposure to infected feces (cat or poultry most commonly in the United States) or by eating undercooked infected meat (beef,

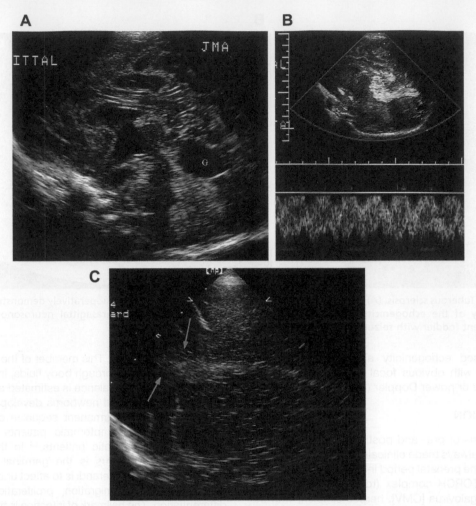

Fig. 17. Vascular malformations. (*A*) Coronal neurosonogram demonstrates a slight increase in the echogenicity of flowing blood in a midline Galenic malformation (G). (*B*) Coronal neurosonogram with duplex Doppler tracing demonstrates exuberant flow about the Galenic malformation. (*C*) Parasagittal neurosonogram through the temporal fossa of a different demonstrates a venous angioma as a focal area of increased echogenicity (*arrows*).

chicken, horse, pig, sheep) or raw vegetables since the resistant oocytes live in the soil. One-third of the world's population is infected. When pregnant women have primary infection, 90% of infants develop bilateral chorioretinitis and half of these infants demonstrate neurologic dysfunction. Basal ganglia and periventricular intracranial calcifications are the most common findings on antenatal imaging.

Rubella infection

Vaccination programs have diminished the number of live cases of rubella infection occurring during pregnancy in the United States, and congenital rubella remains a public health concern worldwide. Rubella syndrome describes infants infected during the first 8 weeks of gestation who are born with cataracts, chorioretinitis, cardiac malformations, deafness, glaucoma, microphthalmia,

and microencephaly. Neurosensory hearing loss is a hallmark. Ultrasound findings include mineralizing vasculopathy, subependymal pseudocysts, debris and strands in the ventricles, migration anomalies, cerebellar hypoplasia, aqueductal stenosis, and delayed myelination. Subependymal pseudocysts are cystlike fluid collections that develop in the germinal matrix due to any insult and are nonspecific for infection (**Fig. 20**).

Herpes simplex infection

Transplacental transmission of herpes simplex virus types 1 and 2 accounts for only about 5% of herpes cases presenting in the neonatal period. The rest are caused by contact with seropositive carriers or infected lesions during or shortly after birth. These infants present for care at the age of 2 to 4 weeks. Infection by herpes simplex in the neonatal period can range from mild to

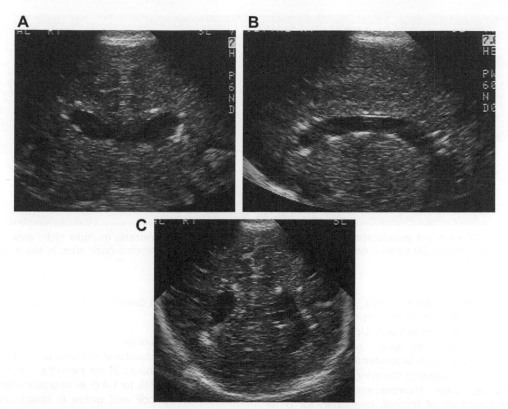

Fig. 18. Periventricular calcifications. (*A*) Anterior coronal neurosonogram demonstrates numerous periventricular calcifications studding the walls of the lateral ventricles in an infant with fetal CMV infection. (*B*) Parasagittal view optimized for the lateral ventricle with subependymal calcifications. (*C*) Posterior coronal view demonstrates additional subependymal calcifications. Similar findings are present in other TORCH infections and in tuberous sclerosis.

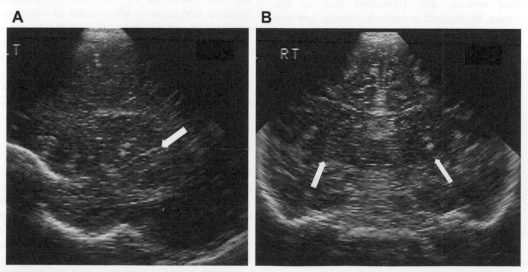

Fig. 19. Mineralizing vasculopathy. (*A*) Parasagittal neurosonogram shows branching echogenic lines of mineral deposits along the lenticulostriate vessels (*arrow*). (*B*) Coronal view demonstrates basal ganglia location of the deposits (*arrows*) medial to the sylvian fissures.

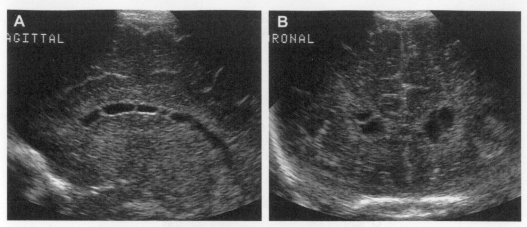

Fig. 20. Subependymal pseudocysts. (*A*) Parasagittal neurosonogram demonstrates multiple cystic areas along the lateral ventricle. (*B*) Coronal neurosonogram demonstrates bilateral symmetric cystic areas in the region of germinal matrix.

disseminated disease. CNS involvement is present in 50%.[30] Presentations include fever, irritability, lethargy, and seizures. Up to 70% of those with CNS infection have encephalitis and mortality, if untreated, is greater than 80%. Neurosonography can detect the congenital anomalies associated with transplacental transmission (same spectrum of findings described for other intrauterine infections) and the brain edema associated with neonatal infection. Heterogeneous appearance of the periventricular white matter or global edema findings of effaced gyral pattern, slit appearance to ventricles, and coarse echo texture should prompt further evaluation with MR imaging and spectroscopy.[31] Other findings that may be seen are hemorrhagic infarction (**Fig. 21**), cerebral edema, and increased flow to the meninges. Multicystic encephalomalacia, cortical

calcification, and cerebral volume loss are long-term sequelae.

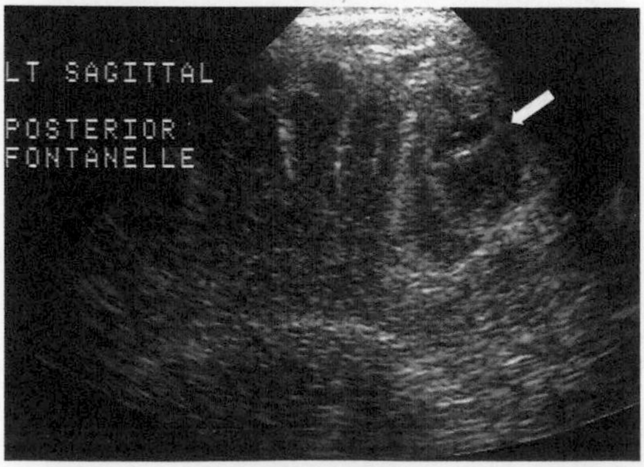

Meningoencephalitis

Clinical signs of bacterial meningitis are minimal when infection occurs in the neonatal period, but prevalence is 1.3% to 1.4% in neonatal intensive care units.[32] *E coli* and group B streptococcus type 3 are common organisms in the neonatal period, and patients often present with seizures and a bulging fontanel. Hemorrhagic meningoencephalitis is usually caused by *Listeria monocytogenes*. More recently, *Bacillus cereus* has been recognized as a cause. Premature male infants are predisposed. Imaging findings include asymmetric areas of increased echogenicity representing focal cerebritis or infarction; porencephaly; cerebral edema with effacement of the cortical markings or coarsening of the echotexture; areas of increased echogenicity equal to or greater than the echogenicity of choroid plexus indicating hemorrhage; increased echogenicity of sulci, meninges, and ventricular walls; and increased echogenicity or complex appearance of the CSF (**Fig. 22**).

INJURY

Prenatal, perinatal, and postnatal injuries cause a spectrum of neurosonographic findings that vary with the maturity of the fetus at the time of the insult. If imaging is used at the suspected time of insult, the findings vary more than the chronic changes seen in the brain after it heals. Unique risks of the preterm infant, perinatal asphyxia, and infants on extracorporeal membrane oxygenation therapy are specifically addressed. Chronic findings are relatively uniform

Fig. 21. Subacute hemorrhagic infarction. Parasagittal image of the left parietal cortex demonstrates an enlarged gyrus with a heterogeneous appearance. Evolving blood products cause a fluid/debris level in the infarct (*arrow*).

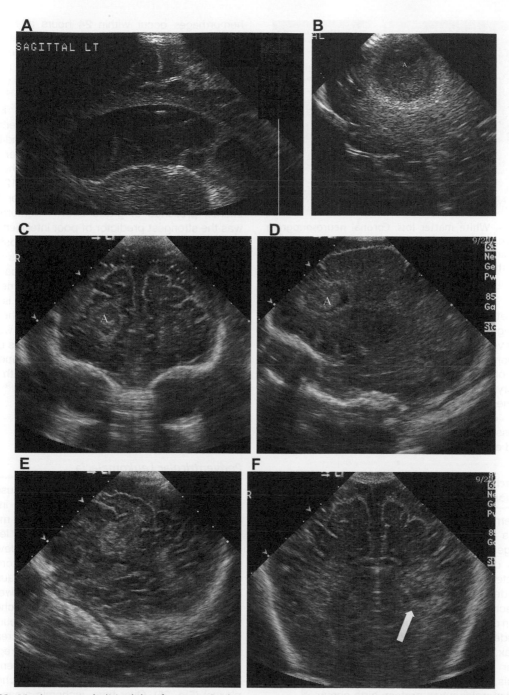

Fig. 22. Meningoencephalitis. (*A*) Left parasagittal neurosonogram demonstrates an enlarged lateral ventricle with increased echogenicity of the ependymal lining, septations, and debris. (*B*) Parasagittal neurosonogram in a different infant demonstrates a complex abscess (A) with surrounding edema. (*C*) Coronal anterior view of a different infant with *Citrobacter* meningitis demonstrates bilateral complex subdural effusions, thickened leptomeninges, cerebritis with increased heterogeneous white matter, and a right frontal abscess (A). (*D*) Right parasagittal view of same patient with *Citrobacter* meningitis demonstrates right frontal abscess (A) and diffuse cerebritis. (*E*) Left parasagittal view of same patient with *Citrobacter* meningitis demonstrates temporal cerebritis with increased heterogeneous gray and white matter. (*F*) Coronal posterior view of same patient with *Citrobacter* meningitis demonstrates diffuse bilateral cerebritis with increased heterogeneous white matter. Note the vague area of liquefaction that is low echogenicity (*arrow*).

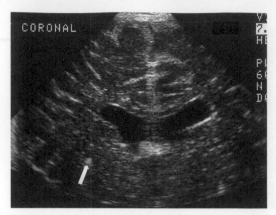

Fig. 23. White matter loss. Coronal neurosonogram demonstrates uniform thinning of the white matter. The sulci are in close proximity to the ventricles. Note the coarse calcification on the right (*arrow*).

no matter what form the initial insult takes. Chronic findings of injury include encephalomalacia, prominent ventricles and extra-axial fluid spaces, calcifications, and atrophy (**Fig. 23**). The presence of any of these findings without an appropriate history of trauma, hypoxia, or infection begs entertainment of nonaccidental trauma as the underlying cause. MR imaging and other clinical assessment tools are used to fully assess the likelihood of abuse.

Intracranial Hemorrhage and Periventricular Hemorrhagic Infarction

Preterm infants are at risk for intracranial hemorrhage because of the rich venous plexus within the germinal matrix before 32 weeks GA. Up to 20% of infants weighing less than 1500 g are affected. Stressors that can lead to hemorrhage include any natural process or therapy that leads to decreased cerebral perfusion followed by restoration of flow with loss of autoregulation. Examples include suctioning of endotracheal tube, pneumothorax, hypotension, and myocardial fatigue. Other independent risk factors include early sepsis, in vitro fertilization, and lack of use of antenatal steroids when preterm birth occurs.[33]

Once hemorrhage occurs, oxygen delivery to the brain is impaired. About 15% of infants with intraventricular hemorrhage develop periventricular hemorrhagic infarctions, which are venous infarctions of the medullary veins in the periventricular white matter.

Because most hemorrhages are clinically silent, screening neurosonography is recommended in all infants of less than 30 weeks GA or with a birth weight of less than 1500 g. Only 30% of

hemorrhages occur within 24 hours after birth, but 90% occur in the first week of life. Unless the infant's clinical condition is deteriorating, delaying the screening examination until days 7 to 14 and once again when the baby reaches 36 to 40 weeks postmenstrual age increases its utility.[34] The grading system of Papile and colleagues[35] is the most widely used system for describing perinatal intraventricular hemorrhage. These conditions range from mild caudothalamic groove germinal matrix bleeds (Grade 1) to periventricular hemorrhagic infarction (Grade 4) (**Fig. 24**). In a 12-year follow-up study of a large cohort of preterm infants, presence of grade 3 or 4 hemorrhage was the strongest predictor of poor intelligence.[36]

Preterm infants are also at risk for posterior fossa hemorrhages that are almost always overlooked if only an anterior fontanelle approach to neurosonography is used. The preferred method for assessing posterior fossa hemorrhage is with the mastoid view (see **Fig. 14**).[37] Once hemorrhage is identified, patients are followed weekly to identify complications like hydrocephalus early. In a recent study, hydrocephalus developed in 21% of patients and was associated with less functional independence at 5 years of age.[38]

Periventricular Leukomalacia

If cerebral blood flow decreases because of inflammation or ischemia in the preterm infant, the immature oligodendroglia of the white matter are at risk for an injury called periventricular leukomalacia. Up to 60% of preterm infants develop neurologic deficits, and periventricular leukomalacia is the most common underlying cause.[39] Factors include sepsis, very low birth weight, younger GA, and cardiac conditions. The ischemic areas may appear completely normal by neurosonography or appear as patchy areas of increased white matter echogenicity, and may have regions of hemorrhagic change (recognized when the abnormal echogenicity is ≥ that of the choroid plexus) (**Fig. 25**). Over time, ischemic areas may fade without long-term neuronal loss or may evolve into regions of porencephalic cyst formation. Cystic periventricular leukomalacia is 1 of 3 major ultrasound findings (the other 2 being Grade 3 or 4 hemorrhage and focal infarction) that were associated with cerebral palsy in high-risk preterm infants.[40] Use of accessory acoustical windows like the mastoid view, posterior fontanelle, and foramen magnum increases the ability to identify areas that are at risk.

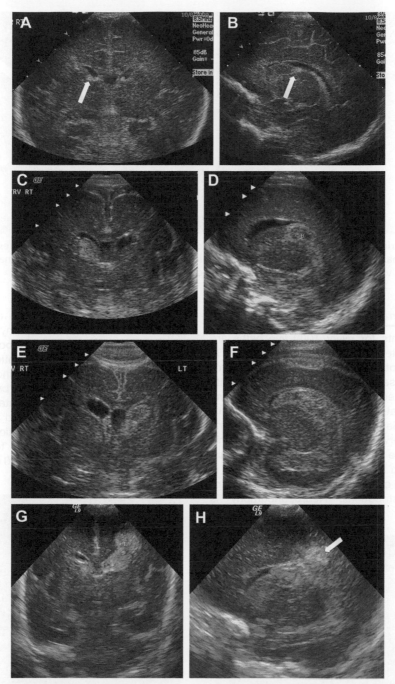

Fig. 24. Intracranial hemorrhage. (*A*) Coronal neurosonogram demonstrates bilateral asymmetric increased echogenicity at the germinal matrix in the caudothalamic groove (*arrow*). (*B*) Left parasagittal view demonstrates the same Grade 1 hemorrhage (*arrow*). (*C*) Coronal neurosonogram on a different preterm infant with echogenic blood within the right lateral ventricle (B). (*D*) Right parasagittal neurosonogram of same infant with Grade 2 hemorrhage (B). (*E*) Coronal neurosonogram from another infant with an enlarged left lateral ventricle filled with blood (B). (*F*) Left parasagittal image shows a "reverse C," which is the blood filling the entire enlarged left lateral ventricle in this Grade 3 hemorrhage. (*G*) Coronal neurosonogram from another preterm infant with blood filling an enlarged left lateral ventricle and an adjacent periventricular hemorrhagic venous infarct (B). (*H*) Left parasagittal image shows the Grade 4 hemorrhage (*arrow*).

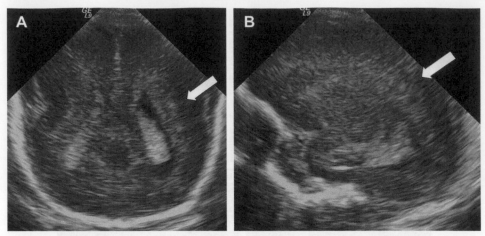

Fig. 25. Periventricular leukomalacia. (*A*) Coronal neurosonogram of a preterm infant with respiratory distress demonstrates small patchy areas of increased echogenicity in the left periventricular white matter (*arrow*). (*B*) Left parasagittal view of the periventricular leukomalacia (*arrow*).

Hypoxic-Ischemic Encephalopathy

Two term infants for every 1000 live births are affected by systemic perinatal asphyxia, and 15% to 20% die. Another 25% have permanent neuropsychological sequelae.[41] Neurologic morbidity has not changed since 1975, although survival rates in these patients have increased. Rapid identification of patients who might benefit from early therapeutic intervention is critical to changing this pattern. The site of involvement in the term infant is different from that in the preterm infant, and is localized in the cerebral cortex within vascular or watershed distributions. Neurosonography is

a poor test for the presence or absence of hypoxic-ischemic encephalopathy and for long-term prognosis.[42] Because the modality is portable and frequently used in unstable patients, it is important to recognize findings that indicate disease. These findings include increased brain echogenicity, coarsening of the brain echotexture, obliteration of the surrounding fluid spaces, and effacement of the convolutional markings (**Fig. 26**). Severe hypoxia leads to increased or decreased resistance indices (<50 or >90), reliably

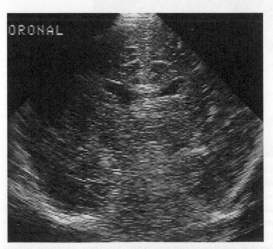

Fig. 26. Cerebral edema. Coronal neurosonogram of an infant who developed brain edema on ECMO. Note the coarse echotexture of the brain, and effacement of the convolutional markings. Contrast with **Fig. 23**.

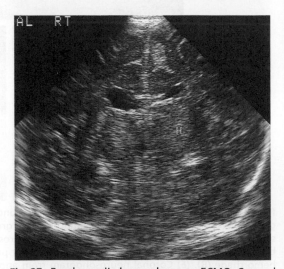

Fig. 27. Basal ganglia hemorrhage on ECMO. Coronal neurosonogram 1 day later than **Fig. 26**. Brain is less edematous as evidenced by the appearance of the convolutional markings. There are isoechoic hemorrhages (H) in the basal ganglia, left larger than right. In the anticoagulated patient, hemorrhage may be isoechoic with brain.

measured with transcranial Doppler. Performance of magnetic resonance imaging, diffusion tensor imaging, and spectroscopy are the gold standards for care in this population.

Extracorporeal Membrane Oxygenation

Extracorporeal Membrane Oxygenation (ECMO) remains a mainstay in the treatment of infants and young adults with respiratory failure. In infancy, conditions that lead to respiratory insufficiency include sepsis, meconium aspiration, pulmonary hypoplasia, and congenital diaphragmatic hernia. A cannula is placed through the right internal jugular vein into the right atrium. Cardiopulmonary bypass allows blood to pass through

the external membrane oxygenator and then returns into the aortic arch through a cannula in the right common carotid artery. Venovenous catheters can also be used so that blood is placed into the right atrium and out of the right atrium. ECMO therapy has a survival rate of 76%, and very high morbidity with severe neurologic disability in 13%.[43] Infants on ECMO are continually anticoagulated and are at risk for intracranial hemorrhage, and for nonhemorrhagic changes in the parenchyma and in the extra-axial fluid spaces that herald future neurologic disability. As long as the fontanelles are open, a baseline sonogram is performed before the placement of the patient on ECMO. Patients are not candidates for ECMO therapy if severe anoxic-ischemic injury, large

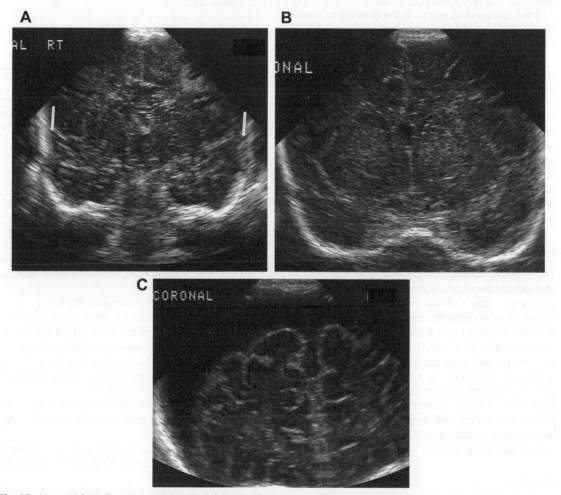

Fig. 28. Nonaccidental trauma spectrum. (*A*) Coronal sonogram demonstrates a left frontotemporal brain contusion that is echogenic. Note the difference in the width of the meninges laterally (*arrows*). The wider meninges on the left are due to subdural hematoma. (*B*) Coronal neurosonogram of a shaken baby demonstrates a wide unsharp appearance to the deep subarachnoid spaces bilaterally, left worse than right. (*C*) Prominent bifrontal extra-axial fluid collections, right worse than left. If there is no history of infection or trauma, consider nonaccidental trauma.

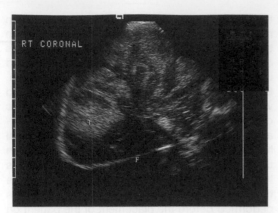

Fig. 29. High-grade astrocytoma. Intraoperative coronal view of the left frontal lobe from a left frontal approach. The falx (F) runs from the vertex on the reader's left to the anterior horns of the lateral ventricles. It is very difficult to differentiate the tumor (T) from surrounding edema at the gray/white matter interface.

infarctions, or intraventricular hemorrhage greater than grade 2 are seen. Daily ultrasound scans are then performed to evaluate the occurrence of hemorrhage. Any hemorrhage above grade 1 is cause for discontinuation of therapy. It should be noted that hemorrhage that occurs while patients are anticoagulated is not as echogenic as hemorrhage that occurs in babies with normal clotting factors. Mass effect that was not seen on the previous sonogram may be the only clue that a hemorrhage has occurred (**Fig. 27**).

Nonaccidental Trauma

The leading cause of morbidity and mortality in abused children is craniocerebral injury. Ultrasound scanning may reveal unexplained subdural effusions or nonspecific cortical findings, and may alert the medical team to the possibility of nonaccidental trauma (**Fig. 28**). The differential diagnosis for unexplained prominence of the subdural CSF is benign macrocrania, where the subarachnoid space over both cerebral convexities is enlarged with normal-sized ventricles, birth trauma, and previous infection. MR imaging is helpful in identifying blood products within the extra-axial fluid when this finding occurs.

TUMOR

Most CNS tumors presenting in infancy are supratentorial (65%) and are most often astrocytomas (30.5%).[44] Solid neoplasms in the brain are most often hyperechoic (**Fig. 29**), and secondary findings of edema and mass effect or hydrocephalus

may also be seen. MR imaging is the gold standard for preoperative imaging. Intraoperative neurosonography continues to play a significant role in care of these infants because extent of resection and histology are the 2 most important prognostic factors.[45,46]

SUMMARY

Neurosonography will continue to be the initial screening modality of choice in infants because of its low cost, portability, and safety. With 3D localization, advances in quantitative algorithms, and forays into ultrasound contrast administration, additional value may be obtained in the future from this bedside modality.

REFERENCES

1. Paladini D, Volpe P. Posterior fossa and vermian morphometry in the characterization of fetal cerebellar abnormalities: a prospective three-dimensional ultrasound study. Ultrasound Obstet Gynecol 2006;27(5):482–9.
2. Padilla NF, Enriquez G, Jansson T, et al. Quantitative tissue echogenicity of the neonatal brain assessed by ultrasound imaging. Ultrasound Med Biol 2009; 35(9):1421–6.
3. He W, Jiang XQ, Wang S, et al. Intraoperative contrast enhanced ultrasound for brain tumors. Clin Imaging 2008;32(6):419–24.
4. Allendoerfer J, Tanislav C. Diagnostic and prognostic value of contrast-enhanced ultrasound in acute stroke. Ultraschall Med 2008;29(Suppl 4): S210–4.
5. Van der Knapp MS, Valk J. Classification of congenital abnormalities of the CNS. AJNR Am J Neuroradiol 1988;9:315.
6. Chaoui R, Benoit B, Mitkowska-Wozniak H, et al. Assessment of intracranial translucency (IT) in the detection of spina bifida at the 11-13-week scan. Ultrasound Obstet Gynecol 2009;34(3):249–52.
7. Hart MN, Malamud N, Ellis WG. The Dandy-Walker syndrome. A clinicopathological study based on 28 cases. Neurology 1972;22:771.
8. Long A, Morgan P, Robson S. Outcome of fetal cerebral posterior fossa anomalies. Prenat Diagn 2006; 26(8):707–10.
9. Patel S, Barkovich AJ. Analysis and classification of cerebellar malformations. AJNR AM J Neuroradiol 2002;23(7):1074–87.
10. Bordarier C, Aicardi J. Dandy-Walker syndrome and agenesis of the cerebellar vermis: diagnostic problems and genetic counselling. Dev Med Child Neurol 1990;32:285.
11. Chadie A, Radi S, Trestard L, et al. Neurodevelopmental outcome in prenatally diagnosed isolated

Neurosonography **531**

agenesis of the corpus callosum. Acta Paediatr 2008;97(4):420–4.

12. Glass HC, Shaw GM, Ma C, et al. Agenesis of the corpus callosum in California 1983-2003: a population-based study. Am J Med Genet A 2008; 146A(19):2495–500.

13. Volpe P, Campobasso G, De Robertis V, et al. Disorders of prosencephalic development. Prenat Diagn 2009;29(4):340–54.

14. Dubourg C, Bendavid C, Pasquier L, et al. Holoprosencephaly. Orphanet J Rare Dis 2007;2(2):8.

15. Hung JH, Shen SH, Guo WY, et al. Prenatal diagnosis of schizencephaly with septo-optic dysplasia by ultrasound and magnetic resonance imaging. J Obstet Gynaecol Res 2008;34(4 Pt 2):674–9.

16. Guerrini R, Marini C. Genetic malformations of cortical development. Exp Brain Res 2006;173(2): 322–33.

17. Byrd SE, Osborn RE, Bohan TP, et al. The CT and MR evaluation of migrational disorders of the brain. Part 1. Lissencephaly and pachygyria. Pediatr Radiol 1989;19(3):151–6.

18. Byrd SE, Osborn RE, Bohan TP, et al. The CT and MR evaluation of migrational disorders of the brain. Part II. Schizencephaly, heterotopia and polymicrogyria. Pediatr Radiol 1989;19(4):219–22.

19. Packard AM, Miller VS, Delgado MR. Schizencephaly: correlations of clinical and radiologic features. Neurology 1997;48(5):1427–34.

20. di Salvo DN. A new view of the neonatal brain: clinical utility of supplemental neurologic US imaging windows. Radiographics 2001;21(4):943–55.

21. Stranzinger E, Huisman TA. Sturge-Weber syndrome. Early manifestations and visualization of disease course. Radiologe 2007;47(12):1126–30.

22. Napolioni V, Curatolo P. Genetics and molecular biology of tuberous sclerosis complex. Curr Genomics 2008;9(7):475–87.

23. Legge M, Sauerbrei E, Macdonald A. Intracranial tuberous sclerosis in infancy. Radiology 1984; 153(3):667–8.

24. Joint Writing Group of the Technology Assessment Committee American Society of Interventional and Therapeutic Neuroradiology, Joint Section on Cerebrovascular Neurosurgery a Section of the American Association of Neurological Surgeons and Congress of Neurological Surgeons; Section of Stroke and the Section of Interventional Neurology of the American Academy of Neurology. Reporting terminology for brain arteriovenous malformation clinical and radiographic features for use in clinical trials. Stroke 2001;32(6):1430–42.

25. Bartels E. Evaluation of arteriovenous malformations (AVMs) with transcranial color-coded duplex sonography: does the location of an AVM influence its sonographic detection? J Ultrasound Med 2005; 24(11):1511–7.

26. Mathiesen T, Peredo I, Edner G, et al. Neuronavigation for arteriovenous malformation surgery by intraoperative three-dimensional ultrasound angiography. Neurosurgery 2007;60(4 Suppl 2):345–50 [discussion: 350–1].

27. Roze E, Kerstjens JM, Maathuis CG, et al. Risk factors for adverse outcome in preterm infants with periventricular hemorrhagic infarction. Pediatrics 2008;122(1):e46–52.

28. Dollard SC, Grosse SD, Ross DS. New estimates of the prevalence of neurological and sensory sequelae and mortality associated with congenital cytomegalovirus infection [review]. Rev Med Virol 2007;17(5):355–63.

29. de Vries LS, Gunardi H, Barth PG, et al. The spectrum of cranial ultrasound and magnetic resonance imaging abnormalities in congenital cytomegalovirus infection. Neuropediatrics 2004; 35(2):113–9.

30. Anzivino E, Fioriti D, Mischitelli M, et al. Herpes simplex virus infection in pregnancy and in neonate: status of art of epidemiology, diagnosis, therapy and prevention. Virol J 2009;6:40.

31. Baskin HJ, Hedlund G. Neuroimaging of herpesvirus infections in children. Pediatr Radiol 2007;37(10): 949–63.

32. Lequin MH, Vermeulen JR, van Elburg RM, et al. *Bacillus cereus* meningoencephalitis in preterm infants: neuroimaging characteristics. AJNR Am J Neuroradiol 2005;26(8):2137–43.

33. Linder N, Haskin O, Levit O, et al. Risk factors for intraventricular hemorrhage in very low birth weight premature infants: a retrospective case-control study. Pediatrics 2003;111(5 Pt 1):e590–5.

34. Ment LR, Bada HS, Barnes P, et al. Practice parameter: neuroimaging of the neonate: report of the Quality Standards Subcommittee of the American Academy of Neurology and the Practice Committee of the Child Neurology Society. Neurology 2002; 58(12):1726–38.

35. Papile J, Burnstein J, Burnstein R, et al. Incidence and evolution of subependymal IVH: a study of infants with birth weights less than 1500 gms. J Pediatr 1978;92:529.

36. Luu TM, Ment LR, Schneider KC, et al. Lasting effects of preterm birth and neonatal brain hemorrhage at 12 years of age. Pediatrics 2009;123(3):1037–44.

37. Sehgal A, El-Naggar W, Glanc P, et al. Risk factors and ultrasonographic profile of posterior fossa haemorrhages in preterm infants. J Paediatr Child Health 2009;45(4):215–8.

38. Vassilyadi M, Tataryn Z, Shamji MF, et al. Functional outcomes among premature infants with intraventricular hemorrhage. Pediatr Neurosurg 2009;45(4): 247–55.

39. Deng W, Pleasure J, Pleasure D. Progress in periventricular leukomalacia. Arch Neurol 2008;65(10):1291–5.

40. De Vries LS, Van Haastert IL, Rademaker KJ, et al. Ultrasound abnormalities preceding cerebral palsy in high-risk preterm infants. J Pediatr 2004;144(6): 815–20.

41. Taniguchi H, Andreasson K. The hypoxic-ischemic encephalopathy model of perinatal ischemia. J Vis Exp 2008;19(21). pii:955. DOI:10.3791/955.

42. Boo NY, Chandran V, Zulfiqar MA, et al. Early cranial ultrasound changes as predictors of outcome during first year of life in term infants with perinatal asphyxia. J Paediatr Child Health 2000;36(4):363–9.

43. Nijhuis-van der Sanden MW, van der Cammen-van Zijp MH, Janssen AJ, et al. Motor performance in five-year-old extracorporeal membrane oxygenation survivors: a population-based study. Crit Care 2009; 13(2):R47.

44. Larouche V, Huang A, Bartels U, et al. Tumors of the central nervous system in the first year of life. Pediatr Blood Cancer 2007;49(Suppl 7):1074–82.

45. Isaacs H Jr. I. Perinatal brain tumors: a review of 250 cases. Pediatr Neurol 2002;27(4):249–61.

46. Isaacs H Jr. II. Perinatal brain tumors: a review of 250 cases. Pediatr Neurol 2002;27(5):333–42.

Transcranial Doppler: Applications in Neonates and Children

Dorothy I. Bulas, MD

KEYWORDS

- Transcranial Doppler • Neurosonology • Pediatric brain
- Neonatal brain • Cranial Doppler sonography
- Resistive index

Duplex Doppler with color flow imaging through the anterior fontanelle is simple and has proved useful in evaluating abnormalities of cerebral blood flow in the neonate.[1–4] Once the fontanelle closes, transcranial Doppler sonography can be performed using a 2- to 2.5-MHz pulsed wave Doppler transducer via the thin temporal bone. First introduced by Aeslid in 1982, this technique can be used to measure the velocity and pulsatility of blood flow within the intracranial arteries of the circle of Willis and the vertebrobasilar system.[5] Transcranial Doppler has become important in the management of children with sickle cell anemia and has proved to be a useful tool in the evaluation of various intracranial pathologies such as asphyxia, hydrocephalus, vascular malformations, vasospasm, and brain death in infants, children, and adults.

There are 2 types of transcranial Doppler equipment: nonimaging (TCD) and imaging (TCDI). Continuous wave and nonimaging pulsed wave Doppler techniques insonate specific vessels using strict criteria for vessel identification based on depth and direction of flow for intracranial vessels via the temporal bone.[6,7] Advantages of this technique include using small, inexpensive, portable units designed specifically for transcranial Doppler, and superior window maneuverability because of small transducer size. Limitations of the nonimaging technique include the need for intensive training, difficulty in finding vessels, and lack of unit availability in many hospitals. Color

Doppler imaging via the anterior fontanelle or transtemporal approach allows for quick vessel identification, resulting in a shorter learning curve, and it is widely available in most radiology departments.[8–10] With training and experience, both techniques have been shown to be reliable with good reproducibility (in the remainder of this article, TCD refers to imaging and nonimaging techniques).[11]

TECHNIQUE
Neonate

In the neonate, the open anterior fontanelle provides an easy approach to insonate the anterior cerebral, middle cerebral, distal internal carotid, and basilar arteries, and the internal cerebral veins, vein of Galen, and superior sagittal sinus. Midline sagittal imaging provides direct insonation of the anterior cerebral artery (ACA) (**Fig. 1A**). The smaller thalamostriate arteries of the middle cerebral artery (MCA) may be visualized on angled sagittal images. On the coronal plane angled anteriorly via the anterior fontanelle, the supraclinoid internal carotid, middle cerebral, thalamostriate, and A1 segment of the anterior cerebral arteries can be visualized (**Fig. 1B**). Angled posteriorly, the internal cerebral veins, thalamostriate arteries, basilar artery, and transverse sinuses can be visualized. As the angle between the middle cerebral arteries and ultrasound beam is often

Department of Diagnostic Imaging and Radiology, Children's National Medical Center, George Washington University Medical Center, 111 Michigan Avenue NW, Washington, DC 20010, USA
E-mail address: dbulas@cnmc.org

Ultrasound Clin 4 (2009) 533–551
doi:10.1016/j.cult.2009.11.001
1556-858X/09/$ – see front matter

ultrasound.theclinics.com

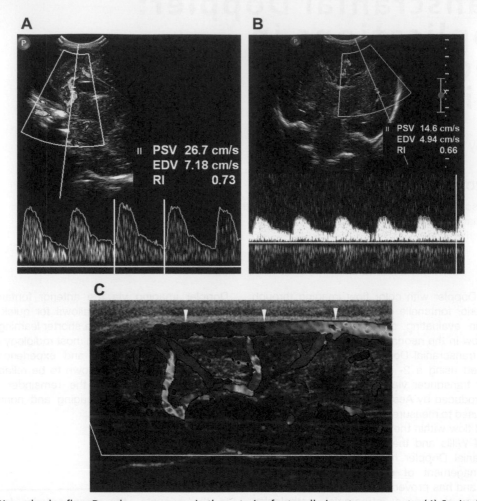

Fig. 1. Normal color flow Doppler sonogram via the anterior fontanelle in a term neonate. (*A*) Sagittal midline view with infant facing the left demonstrates the ACA coursing over the corpus callosum. Cursor is placed on the pericallosal artery demonstrating a normal RI for a term infant measuring 0.73. (*B*) Coronal view with cursor placed on the peripheral left MCA demonstrating a normal RI of 0.66. (*C*) Sagittal view using a linear transducer demonstrates flow in small cortical veins draining into the superior sagittal sinus (*arrowheads*).

perpendicular in this plane, frequency shifts can approach zero and Doppler signal is thus poor.

Proper technique includes adjusting color gain to maximize vascular signal and minimize tissue motion artifacts. The lowest band pass filter should be used to maximize low flow sensitivity when evaluating venous structures. Linear 7- to 15-MHz transducers are particularly useful in evaluating the sagittal sinus and vessels crossing the subarachnoid space (**Fig. 1**C).

Child

Once the anterior fontanelle closes, 3 cranial windows are available to insonate the intracranial circulation: the temporal bone, the orbit, and the foramen magnum.[12] The transtemporal approach is via the thin suprazygomatic portion of the

temporal bone using a 2- to 3-MHz transducer cephalad to the zygomatic arch, anterior to the ear. On gray-scale imaging the heart-shaped cerebral peduncles are a useful landmark for identification. Anterior to the peduncles is the echogenic suprasellar cistern, where the circle of Willis lies. The MCA is seen as a vessel coursing toward the transducer (**Fig. 2**A). Deeper toward the midline, the bifurcation of the A1 ACA and the MCA can be identified with bidirectional flow (flow toward the transducer in the MCA and flow in the ACA away from the transducer [**Fig. 2**B]). As the transducer is angled anteriorly, flow from the ACA courses away from the transducer. The distal internal cerebral artery is inferior to the bifurcation with lower flow velocities than the MCA because of the larger angle of insonation. The posterior cerebral artery (PCA) is visualized as it circles around

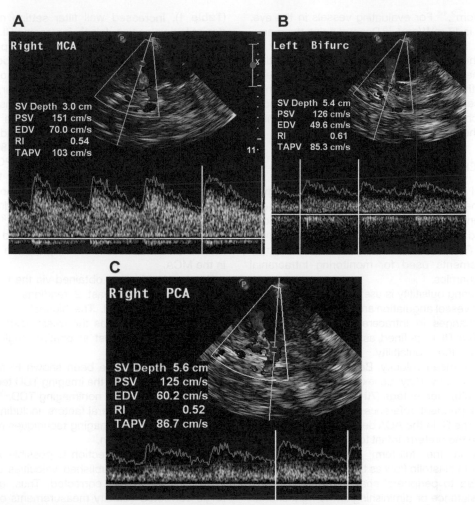

Fig. 2. Transtemporal window. (*A*) Transtemporal color flow Doppler image shows the circle of Willis anterior to the cerebral peduncles. Cursor is placed on the distal MCA with flow directed toward the transducer in red. PSV, EDV, RI, and time average maximum mean velocity (TAMMX /TAMX/TAPV) are recorded. (*B*) Bifurcation of MCA and ACA with flow toward transducer in red the MCA and away from transducer in blue the ACA. (*C*) Cursor placed on the PCA with flow directed toward the transducer. The PCA courses around the cerebral peduncles, which appear heart shaped.

the cerebral peduncles first coursing toward then away from the transducer (**Fig. 2**C). The contralateral MCA, ACA, and PCA, at times, may also be visualized.[13]

The vertebral and basilar arteries are insonated via the foramen magnum. The patient lies on 1 side or prone with the head bent. The transducer is placed midline and angled through the foramen magnum toward the orbits. The vertebral arteries appear V-shaped as they form the basilar artery between the hypoechoic medulla-pons junction and the echogenic clivus. Flow in the vertebral and basilar arteries should be directed away from the transducer.

SAFETY

Energy is imparted into tissues during pulsed wave and color flow Doppler examinations. Although transcranial Doppler ultrasound is considered safe, biologic effects may be identified in the future. "As low as reasonably achievable" (ALARA) principles should be used, with Doppler exposure time limited, and signal intensity maximized by increasing gain rather than transducer power output settings. The American Institute of Ultrasound and Medicine and the US federal guidelines of the spatial peak time averaged intensity (I_{SPTA}) for the pediatric head recommend not exceeding

94 mW/cm^2.[14] For evaluating vessels in the eye, the limit is 17 mW/cm^2.[15] Depending on the manufacturer and transducer, energy levels may be within the guidelines only on low power setting. When the transtemporal approach is used, at least 65% of the energy is attenuated by the skull. Thus, higher settings may be used via the transtemporal approach but should not be exceeded when insonating the eye or foramen magnum.[16]

DOPPLER MEASUREMENTS

Spectral analysis of the waveform can display many measurements. The peak systolic velocity (PSV), end diastolic velocity (EDV), resistive index (RI), and time average mean of the maximum velocity (TAMMX/TAP/TAM) are the most common measurements used for monitoring intracranial hemodynamics.

Measuring pulsitility is useful as it minimizes the effect of vessel angulation and correlates well with acute changes in intracerebral perfusion pressure.[4] The RI is defined as the PSV−EDV/PSV, whereas the pulsitility index (PI) equals PSV−EDV/mean velocity. Because the RI and PI are ratios, they may be expressed as a whole number (70), percentage (70%), or fraction (0.7).

Age-dependent reference values are available for RIs. The RI in the ACA decreases from a mean of 0.79 in the preterm infant to a mean of 0.7 (range 0.6–0.8) in the full-term newborn.[3,17–19] The increase in diastolic flow as the neonate ages may be related to peripheral changes in cerebrovascular resistance or diminishing left to right shunts. Although published normal velocities are broad in the neonate, variability in an individual infant should not be large, with changes of more than 50% from baseline values considered abnormal. There should not be significant differences in pulsitility among the ACA, MCA, PCA, or right and left branches if the circle of Willis is patent. By age 2 years, the normal RI is 0.5 ± 15% (range 0.43–0.58).[4,20]

The ophthalmic artery (OA) is an exception with a higher RI (usually 0.70–0.79) and less diastolic flow as it supplies muscular beds.[12]

An increase in diastolic flow results in a decrease in the RI, whereas a decrease in diastolic flow results in an increase in the RI. As intracranial pressure (ICP) increases more than mean arterial pressure, diastolic flow may become reversed, demonstrating an RI of greater than 1.[20]

Various factors can influence resistive indices. Left to right shunts such as patent ductus arteriosus (PDA) and scanning pressure on the anterior fontanelle can increase RI, whereas tachycardia or decreased cardiac output can decrease RI

(Table 1). Increased wall filter setting may not depict low velocities, falsely increasing RI.

Although easy to obtain, RI is a weak predictor of cerebrovascular resistance, with blood flow velocity measures more informative. To obtain accurate velocity measurements, however, appropriate cursor placement and angle of insonation are critical. Normal mean velocities slowly decrease through puberty, and by adulthood velocities in the MCA range from 50 to 80 cm/s, in the ACA from 35 to 60 cm/s, in the PCA from 30 to 50 cm/s, and in the basilar artery from 25 to 50 cm/s. Peak systolic velocities more than 150 cm/s have been described in children with sickle cell disease secondary to anemia.[21,22] The velocity in the PCA and vertebral and basilar arteries should be approximately half the velocity in the MCA.

When velocities are obtained via the transtemporal approach, at least 2 readings should be made for each vessel. The highest velocity obtained may be taken as the truest velocity, as it is likely to be the best insonating angle to the vessel.[16]

Peak velocities have been shown to measure 5% to 10% lower with the imaging TCD technique (TCDI) compared with nonimaging TCD.[23,24] This may be related to several factors, including larger transducer size with imaging techniques resulting in larger angle variation.

Although angle correction is possible with the imaging technique, published velocities typically have not been angle corrected. Thus, although angle-corrected velocity measurements obtained with the imaging technique may be more accurate than nonangle-corrected velocity measurements, in clinical applications such as assessing stroke risk in children with sickle cell anemia, guidelines regarding normal versus abnormal/conditional velocities were validated in large clinical trials using nonduplex equipment that were not angle corrected.[23–29]

There are many pitfalls when performing a transcranial Doppler examination in neonates and children.[29–31] Low wall filter adjustments, high Doppler frequency, and critical assessment of velocity spectral analysis are important for accurate interpretation.[10] Although a patent circle of Willis can be assumed in children, 1 artery tracing should not be used to represent the entire cerebral circulation evaluation.

ABNORMAL CEREBRAL HEMODYNAMICS

Cerebral hemodynamics are affected by numerous factors. In neonates, high peak inspiratory pressures have been shown to decrease

Table 1
Cerebral Doppler pulsitility changes

	Resistive Index
Intracranial Abnormalities	
Intracranial bleed	Increased
PVL	Increased
Cerebral edema	Increased
Hydrocephalus	Increased, increases with fontanelle pressure, normalizes (decreases) after drainage
Subdural hemorrhage	Increased
Brain death	Increased (then no flow)
Asphyxia	Decreased initially (then increases as edema develops)
ECMO	Decreased
Vascular malformations	Decreased
Extracranial Abnormalities	
P_{CO_2}	Inversed (increased CO_2 = decreased RI)
Heart rate	Inversed (increased HR = decreased RI)
PDA	Increased
Pneumothorax	Increased
Cardiac ischemia	Increased
Polycythemia	Increased
Anemia	Increased
Medications	
Indomethacin	Increased
Surfactant	Increased

Abbreviations: ECMO, extracorporeal membrane oxygenation; PDA, patent ductus arteriosus; PVL, periventricular leukomalacia.

venous return with resultant reversal of intracranial venous flow.[32] Endotracheal suctioning can increase mean arterial blood pressure in premature infants with impaired cerebral blood flow autoregulation.[33] Extracorporeal membrane oxygenation with cannulation of the right common carotid artery and jugular vein results in decreased pulsitility of the intracranial vessels.

Medications such as indomethacin, anemia, changes in CO_2 (sleeping increases CO_2, hyperventilation decreases CO_2), and the presence of arteriovenous malformations/PDA can alter cerebral hemodynamics and also need to be taken into account (see **Table 1**).

Indications

Subarachnoid versus subdural collections
Color flow Doppler using high frequency linear transducers can be used to differentiate subarachnoid fluid from subdural collections. Superficial cortical blood vessels lie between the pia and arachnoid. Fluid in the subarachnoid space lifts the cortical vessels away from the brain surface (**Fig. 3**). Fluid in the subdural space pushes cortical vessels toward the brain surface (**Fig. 4**).[34] Infants may present with asymptomatic macrocephaly caused by disproportionate growth of the calvarium compared with the brain. This transient condition usually resolves spontaneously. Extra-axial fluid may be difficult to distinguish on computed tomography (CT) as subarachnoid versus subdural, particularly if the subdural fluid is subacute or chronic and of low density. Thus, normal subarachnoid fluid can be distinguished from subdural fluid using Doppler to identify crossing vessels.

Venous thrombosis
Venous sinus thrombosis can develop secondary to dehydration, coagulopathy, or infection. Although phase-contrast magnetic resonance (MR) venography is the imaging modality of choice, neonates too unstable for an MR examination may be evaluated by Doppler via the anterior fontanelle. Venous flow may be absent or

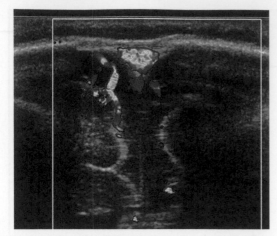

Fig. 3. Subarachnoid fluid. Coronal view via the anterior fontanelle demonstrates flow in the superior sagittal sinus. Subarachnoid fluid surrounds and lifts small cortical blood vessels from the surface of the brain. These vessels are crossing the subarachnoid space.

nonocclusive thrombi noted.[33] Venous infarctions of the parasagittal, thalamic, and temporal lobes may develop because of sagittal sinus, straight sinus/vein of Galen, and vein of Labbé thromboses. Up to 25% of venous infarcts may become hemorrhagic. Treatment is typically supportive although anticoagulation therapy has been suggested.

Vascular malformations
Transcranial Doppler can be useful for characterizing vascular malformations in the unstable neonate.[3,35] Vascular malformations may present

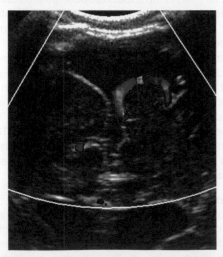

Fig. 4. Subdural fluid. Coronal view via the anterior fontanelle demonstrates cortical vessels compressed against the brain surface. There are no vessels crossing the extra-axial fluid.

with high-output congestive heart failure, hydrocephalus, seizures, or hemorrhage. Spectral analysis reveals turbulent flow with high mean and peak systolic velocities, and low pulsatility caused by increased diastolic flow.

Color flow Doppler imaging can characterize the type of vein of Galen malformation. The choroidal type is characterized by multiple abnormal feeding vessels in the midbrain that drain via a dilated vein of Galen and straight sinus. The infundibular type is an arteriovenous fistula with 1 or a few arterial feeders that directly feed into the vein of Galen. Transcranial Doppler can correctly diagnose arteriovenous malformations with a sensitivity of 87% to 95%.[36–39] Because MR imaging (MRI) has a higher sensitivity in diagnostic screening, Doppler imaging is most useful for quantitating the hemodynamics and monitoring the effects of surgical or vascular interventions (**Fig. 5**).[40] After surgery or embolization, the decrease in systolic velocity and increase in RI of the feeding arteries can be monitored.

Transcranial Doppler has also been used to assess other vascular anomalies such as Sturge-Weber syndrome and dural arteriovenous fistulas.[41,42] Decreased arterial flow velocity and increased PI have been noted with Sturge-Weber syndrome, suggesting chronic hypoperfusion of the tissue to that region.

Hydrocephalus
The ability to differentiate between ventriculomegaly and hydrocephalus (ventriculomegaly caused by increased intracranial pressure) can be difficult. When hydrocephalus develops, ICP increases, resulting in a decrease in diastolic flow. Stable ventriculomegaly should have normal pulsatility. Increased RI in patients in whom ventricular size is increased may imply increased ICP and the need for a shunt. Because TCD is portable, noninvasive, safe, and repeatable, Doppler can be used to assess changes in cerebral hemodynamics in hydrocephalus through the anterior fontanelle in infants and through the temporal bone in older children.[4,43,44] Experimental fontanometric and direct measurement evidence has shown a direct correlation between ICP and RI, caused by a reduction in EDV.[44,45]

Because the volume of brain, cerebrospinal fluid (CSF) and blood is constant, during graded fontanelle compression, CSF or blood should normally be displaced to compensate for small increases in volume with no change in ICP. In infants with hydrocephalus, the increase in volume with compression translates into a transient increase in ICP with an acute increase in arterial pulsatility. Serial examinations can follow the infant's ability

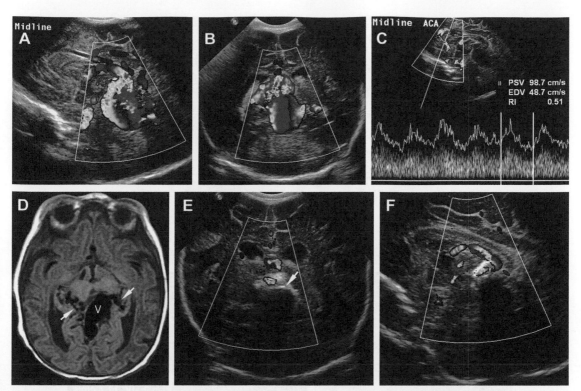

Fig. 5. Vein of Galen aneurysm in a newborn infant presenting with congestive heart failure. (*A*) Sagittal and (*B*) coronal views via the anterior fontanelle show a large dilated vein of Galen aneurysm. (*C*) Sagittal pulsed Doppler tracing of the pericallosal artery demonstrates abnormal high peak and end diastolic velocities with a dampened pulsitility. (*D*) Axial T1w MR images confirms the presence of a large vein of Galen aneurysm (V) with arterial feeders (*arrows*). Postembolization (*E*) sagittal and (*F*) coronal images demonstrate successful occlusion of the feeding vessels with shadowing in the vicinity of the vein of Galen secondary to coil placement (*arrow*). The infant did well following intervention.

to compensate for minor changes in intracranial volume.

Pulsatility drops following ventricular tapping and shunting in infants with hydrocephalus.[11,46] Taylor[47,48] directly measured changes in ICP before and after ventricular drainage procedures and correlated this with changes in RI (**Fig. 6**). Increased ICP, however, is not always present in infants with ventricular dilation. Doppler during fontanelle compression may be useful in the early identification of infants with abnormal intracranial compliance before the development of increased ICP.[47,49] With fontanelle compression, Taylor showed that changes in RI can be a strong predictor of increased ICP and can help identify who would benefit from shunt placement (**Fig. 7**).[48] This technique has also been used to evaluate intracranial compliance in young children with craniosynostosis before repair.[50]

There are 2 major problems with using RI.[51] First, other intracranial and extracranial factors besides increased ICP can change the RI (see **Table 1**). Thus, the RI must be correlated with the clinical condition of the patient (eg, Pco_2, heart

rate, PDA). Second, there is a range of normal values (0.65–0.85 in the neonate; 0.60–0.70 in the child before fontanelle closure; 0.50–0.60 in older children and adults). Goh and colleagues[44] used an RI of greater than 0.8 as a sign of increased pressure in the neonate and an RI of greater than 0.65 in children. As there is a wide variation of normal and an overlap between normal and abnormal values, RI is most useful on an individual basis following a patient's course to determine whether clinical changes or ventricular dilation are secondary to increased pressure or atrophy.

TCD can be used for predicting shunt malfunction, with an increase in RI suggesting shunt malfunction. False normal values, however, may be the result of CSF fluid tracking along the shunt. Excessive thickness of the skull may prevent TCD from being obtained successfully in some of these older patients.[52,53]

Asphyxia

Mild asphyxia typically does not alter cerebral hemodynamics. In the setting of severe or

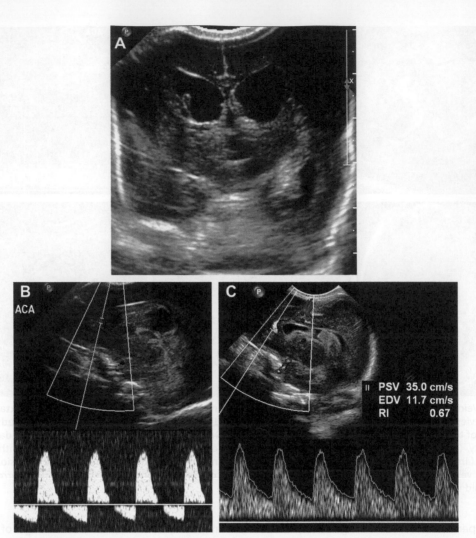

Fig. 6. Two-week-old infant with hydrocephalus secondary to intraventricular hemorrhage. (*A*) Coronal image demonstrates moderate dilatation of the lateral and third ventricles. (*B*) Pulsed Doppler tracing of the ACA documents markedly pulsatile flow with reversal of flow in diastole. (*C*) Following repeated ventricular taps, resistive indices normalized with stabilization of hydrocephalus.

prolonged asphyxia, however, hypoxic injury results in release or decreased reuptake of glutamate and aspartate with production of intracellular nitric oxide with resultant cerebral vasodilatation.[54] Asphyxia may impair cerebral autoregulation, producing an increase in diastolic blood flow and a decrease in cerebrovascular resistance and pulsitility (**Fig. 8**).[2]

TCD may be useful for determining which premature infants are at risk for intraventricular hemorrhage or periventricular leukomalacia (PVL). Blankenberg and colleagues[55] demonstrated that premature infants with germinal matrix hemorrhage had a greater mean velocity and lower RIs in the lenticulostriate vessels.

Intracranial Doppler imaging in the term neonate has been useful in predicting significant

hypoxic-ischemic brain injury.[1,55–59] Archer and colleagues[58] and Stark and Seibert[56] reported a strong correlation with low RI <0.60 and adverse neurologic outcome when performed within the first 48 hours of the insult. The finding of increased diastolic flow can also be useful in evaluating the older child after head injury or cardiac arrest to predict significant cerebral injury before CT findings.

Trauma

Head trauma initiates several pathologic processes that change cerebral hemodynamics, the knowledge of which can be useful for guiding appropriate management. Following a significant cerebral hypoxic insult, vasodilatation may occur, with increase in diastolic flow velocity and reduced

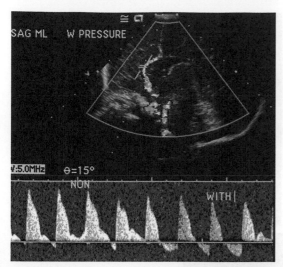

Fig. 7. Effect of increased fontanelle pressure on RI in an infant with hydrocephalus. Pulsed wave Doppler tracing of the ACA, initially with the transducer held lightly over the anterior fontanelle then with compression, demonstrates a further increase in RI with reversal of flow in diastole during compression indicating abnormal intracranial compliance. (*Courtesy of* Richard Barth, MD, Stanford Medical Center, Stanford, CA.)

RI during this early hyperemic phase. As ICP increases, the diastolic flow velocity decreases, with a spike pattern appearance of the PSV. As cerebral edema develops, there is further loss of diastolic flow with reversal in diastole (**Fig. 9**).[45] Continuous or intermittent sequential TCD following a cerebral insult can be helpful in evaluating the presence of edema and the course of treatment.[60]

Treatment of cerebral edema includes hyperventilation. There is an inverse relationship between P_{CO_2} and the RI; the higher the P_{CO_2}, the greater the vasodilatation with increased diastolic flow and lower RI. When the P_{CO_2} is decreased, there is vasoconstriction with a decrease in diastolic flow and increased RI. CO_2 reactivity can be measured following changes in RI. The cerebral blood flow has been shown to increase 4% per mm Hg increase in CO_2.[1,45,59,61] The absence of change in the RI as a patient is being hyperventilated (absent "CO_2 reactivity test") is a sign of severe brain injury.[61] RI is thus useful in monitoring hyperventilation therapy following head trauma.[2,62] As hyperventilation decreases the P_{CO_2}, the RI should increase with vasoconstriction of cerebral vessels. Increasing cerebral edema also increases the RI. Therefore, changes in RI need to be correlated with other clinical findings.

Brain death

Establishing brain death can be problematic, with rapid confirmation important in cases for organ transplant donation. Neurologic examination, electroencephalogram (EEG), and brain stem-evoked potential can be used to establish brain death. Nuclear brain flow studies can be used to determine brain death also, but require transportation of the unstable patient to the nuclear medicine department. TCD is another noninvasive tool that can help assess supratentorial cerebral perfusion. For patients in phenobarbital coma in which an EEG is not diagnostic, TCD is particularly helpful in demonstrating the severity of cerebrovascular compromise.[63-65]

Following a severe asphyxiating event, there may be an initial drop in RI caused by intracranial vasodilation. As cerebral edema develops, there is loss of forward diastolic flow followed by reversal of diastolic flow if ICP exceeds mean arterial pressure, which results in an increase in RI measuring greater than 1 as diastolic flow reverses. Eventually, cerebral blood flow arrest begins to develop at the microcirculation level (see **Fig. 9**). Large vessels distend, then constrict, and eventually thrombose or collapse. As ICP further increases more than mean arterial pressure, arrest of large vessel cerebral circulation results in a decrease in antegrade systolic velocity. Small early systolic spikes and complete arrest of antegrade flow occurs (**Fig. 10**). Finally, no systolic or diastolic flow can be detected.[64,66]

There is some concern about the reliability of TCD in assessing infant brain death. Conditions outside the cranium that are reversible can increase the RI more than 1 in the neonate, such as PDA.[4,67] In neonates, low RIs have been described in patients clinically dead, whereas infants with high RIs have survived.[67,68]

After fontanelle closure, sustained reversal of diastolic flow is characteristic of absent effective cerebral flow in the adult and older child (**Box 1**).[68-70] Studies have demonstrated that TCD waveforms with absent or reversed diastolic flow or small early systolic spikes in at least 2 intracranial arteries are present with brain death but not with patients in coma.[66,71] There are a few pediatric cases of mild diastolic reversed flow that demonstrated recovery of forward diastolic flow and brain stem function.[70,71] Kirkham[63] suggested using a direction of flow index (DFI = 1−maximum diastolic velocity area/maximum systolic velocity area). In his study, all children with substantial diastolic reversed flow and a time average velocity of less than 10 cm/s for a 30-minute period died. A series by Qian[72] found that in children reversed diastolic flow, small systolic forward flow, or

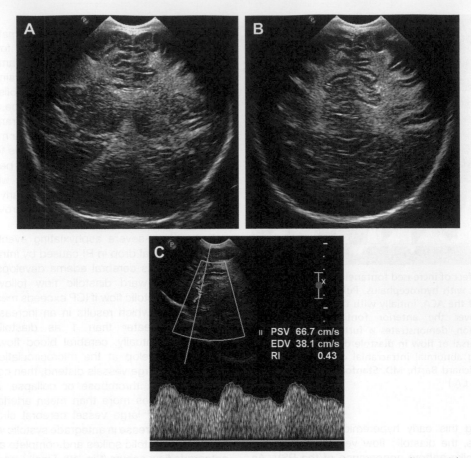

Fig. 8. Severe perinatal asphyxia in a newborn infant. (*A, B*) Coronal images demonstrate slit ventricles and tight sulci consistent with diffuse edema. (*C*) Pulsed Doppler tracing of the ACA demonstrates increased flow during diastole with a low RI measuring 0.43.

a DFI less than 0.8 in the MCA for more than 2 hours was a reliable indicator to confirm brain death.

Undetectable flow in the brain has been described in brain death.[70–73] The occurrence of undetectable middle cerebral flow, however, could be caused by technical factors or distorted anatomy following trauma. The use of contrast agents may improve the level of confidence when no flow is encountered.

Feri and colleagues[71] described 3 waveform patterns in the MCA and extracranial internal carotid and vertebral arteries that were specific for brain death: (1) diastolic reverse flow without systolic forward flow, (2) brief systolic forward flow, and (3) undetectable flow. Their series found that absence of middle cerebral flow on TCD with a simultaneous reversal of diastolic flow in the extracranial internal carotid artery was a reliable sign of cerebral circulatory arrest. A study by Jalili and colleagues[74] reported 100% specificity for brain death when bilateral reversal of diastolic

flow in the internal carotid artery of children was identified.

The TCD examination should never be used in isolation because the arrest of supratentorial flow is not synonymous with brain death. TCD assessment helps indicate the severity of cerebrovascular arrest and should be used as an adjunct confirmatory test, not the sole examination.[75]

Vasospasm

Transcranial Doppler is often used in imaging vasospasm after subarachnoid hemorrhage in adults. It is specific (98–100%)[76,77] in the diagnosis of vasospasm after subarachnoid hemorrhage following rupture of an intracranial aneurysm.[78,79] The vasospasm usually develops in the first 2 days after the hemorrhage, slowly increases (peaking between 11 and 17 days), before gradually decreasing. Patients with persistent severe vasospasm may develop permanent deficits caused by cerebral infarction. Blood flow velocity increases because of a decrease in the

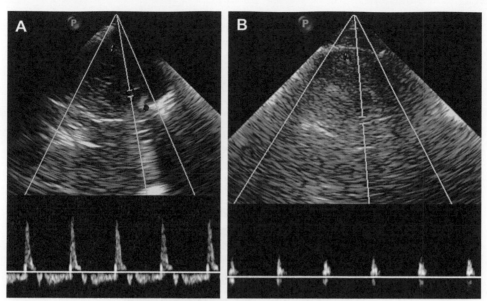

Fig. 9. Two-year-old child following severe traumatic brain injury from a fall. (*A*) Pulsed Doppler tracing 1 day post injury demonstrates abnormal low velocity systolic spikes with reversal of diastolic flow. (*B*) At follow-up, 1 day later, systolic velocities have markedly decreased with no diastolic flow evolving to a brain death pattern.

luminal cross-sectional area of the affected vessels. Thus, TCD can be used to guide optimal timing of therapy before neurologic deficits develop and can be used to follow the effects of therapies. When a hemodynamically significant vasospasm of clinical concern is suggested, balloon dilation angioplasty or intra-arterial infusion of vasodilating agents can be attempted.[80] Serial TCD studies showing reduction in velocities can help determine appropriate time to withdraw therapy, shortening the stay in the intensive care unit. TCD is most accurate in predicting vasospasm of the MCA and is not useful in assessing the ACA beyond its A1 segment or distal MCA branches.

In assessing vasospasm in adults, peak systolic velocities of the MCA have been shown to be most accurate. A PSV of 100 to 140 cm/s correlates with mild vasospasm, velocities of 140 to 200 cm/s correlate with moderate vasospasm, and severe vasospasm is defined as PSV greater than 200 cm/s (**Fig. 11**). A steep increase (>25 cm/s/d) in velocity in the first few days after subarachnoid hemorrhage has been associated with a poorer prognosis. As velocities at baseline may be higher in children, sequential monitoring of velocities is more important in the assessment of vasospasm in this age group.

Sources of error in the detection of vasospasm by TCD (compared with arteriography) include missing peripheral vasospasm, presence of increased ICP, low volume flow, and abnormal baseline velocities.[7] Thus, TCD values should always be combined with clinical and laboratory data.[81,82]

Cerebral vasculitis (small vessel vasculopathy) presenting with stroke is uncommon in children, but does occur from various causes (postinfectious, autoimmune, and idiopathic). Vascular changes are best characterized with MR angiography (MRA) and angiography. Aggressive therapy to prevent further stroke may include high-dose steroids or cyclophosphamide. As progression of stroke or recurrent stroke is the only measure of failure of therapy or progression of disease, it can be useful to monitor these children with TCD sequentially between MRA and catheter angiogram procedures. TCD in these patients may identify early cerebrovascular changes that may require further evaluation and intervention, possibly before the onset of further strokes.[80]

Headaches

Adults with vascular headaches have been evaluated by TCD.[7] Headaches caused by increased ICP may demonstrate abnormal pulsitility.[83] In patients with migraine, a study by Thie[83] found a significant increase in mean velocity compared with controls during headache-free periods. Patients with common migraines had decreased intracranial velocities and increased pulsatility during headache attacks, whereas patients with classic migraines demonstrated an increase in velocities and a decrease in pulsitility (**Fig. 12**).[84]

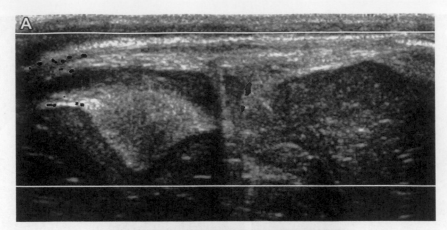

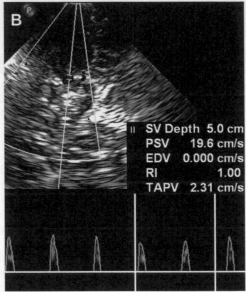

SV Depth 5.0 cm
PSV   19.6 cm/s
EDV   0.000 cm/s
RI   1.00
TAPV   2.31 cm/s

Fig. 10. Nine-month-old infant following nonaccidental trauma. (*A*) Coronal image via the anterior fontanelle demonstrates extra-axial echogenic material overlying the right convexity consistent with subdural hemorrhage, confirmed by CT scan. No significant peripheral arterial or venous flow is documented. (*B*) Transtemporal color Doppler images demonstrate no flow within the circle of Willis. Pulsed Doppler tracing of the distal internal carotid artery demonstrates low velocity spikes in systole with no diastolic flow.

In their series of children with isolated headaches, Wang and colleagues[85] reported the sensitivity and specificity of TCD in detecting intracranial lesions was 75% and 99.7%, respectively.

Sickle cell disease
In children with sickle cell disease, anemia decreases viscosity and increases flow rate. Cerebral infarction secondary to occlusive vasculopathy is a major complication of children with sickle cell disease, with a prevalence ranging from 5.5% to 17%.[86,87] The stenotic lesions typically involve large vessels of the distal internal, proximal middle, and anterior cerebral artery circulation, and progress for months and years

before symptoms develop. Prevention of stroke symptoms by hypertransfusion therapy and bone marrow transplantation in children at risk can lead to stabilization of vasculopathy.[88,89] TCD has proved to be a safe, reliable, and cost-effective screening method to identify children at risk.

Adams and colleagues[21,22,88,90,91] first showed the effectiveness of nonimaging Doppler imaging in screening for cerebrovascular disease in sickle cell disease. Using the nonimaging technique via the transtemporal approach, he found that a mean flow velocity in the MCA equal to or greater than 170 cm/s was an indicator of a patient at risk for development of stroke. Comparing TCD with cerebral angiography, these investigators noted 5

<table>
<tr><td>

Box 1
TCD criteria for brain death after fontanelle closure

Sustained reversal of diastolic flow

Small early systolic spikes

No flow in the MCA with reversal of diastolic flow in the extracranial ICA

Mean velocity in the MCA of less than 10 cm/s for more than 30 minutes

</td></tr>
</table>

criteria for cerebrovascular disease: (1) TAMMX mean velocity of 190 cm/s, (2) low velocity in the MCA (<70 cm/s), (3) MCA ratio of 0.5 or less, (4) ACA/MCA ratio greater than 1.2 on the same side, and (5) inability to detect an MCA in the presence of a demonstrated ultrasound window.[91] Using duplex Doppler imaging, MRA, and MRI, Seibert and colleagues described 9 indicators of cerebrovascular disease in sickle cell patients: (1) maximum velocity in the OA of more than 35 cm/s; (2) TAMMX mean velocity in the MCA of more than 170 cm/s; (3) RI in the OA less than 0.6; (4) velocity in the OA greater than that of the ipsilateral MCA; (5) maximum velocity in the PCA, vertebral, or basilar arteries greater than maximum velocity in the MCA; (6) turbulence; (7) PCA or ACA visualized without seeing the MCA; (8) any RI less than 0.3; and (9) maximum MCA velocity greater than 200 cm/s.[92]

The STOP (Stroke Prevention Trial in Sickle Cell Anemia) study led by Adams[88,93–95] showed that regular transfusion of children at risk for stroke, as determined by Doppler, could prevent stroke. Adams studied 130 children, aged 2 to 16 years, who were at risk to develop stroke, with TAMMX mean velocity in the MCA greater than 200 cm/s. Half received blood transfusions every 3 to 4 weeks. After 1 year, the transfusions lowered the stroke risk by 90%. Patients with a mean velocity greater than 200 cm/s or a PSV greater than 250 cm/s on 2 examinations are recommended for hypertransfusion therapy to prevent stroke (**Table 2**).[96] Correlation with MRI and MRA findings is useful in these patients. Children with abnormal TCD and abnormal MRI are at higher risk for developing a new silent infarct or stroke than those with an abnormal TCD but normal MRI.[97,98]

Screening a patient with sickle cell disease with either the nonimaging or imaging duplex Doppler technique requires scanning the patient transtemporally to evaluate the MCA, bifurcation, distal ICA, ACA, and PCA. The peak systolic, end diastolic, TAMMX, and RI of each of these vessels should be measured at least twice. The MCA should be tracked from the peripheral branch to the bifurcation, obtaining velocities every 2 mm.[93]

When assigning the risk of stroke based on TAMMX it is important to consider how velocities may differ with the imaging equipment compared with nonimaging equipment in the initial STOP studies. Nonangle-corrected velocities obtained with the imaging technique have been shown to be approximately 10% lower in the MCA than those obtained with the nonimaging technique.[23–25] Other studies have shown no

A

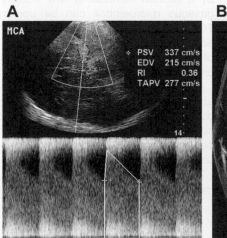

B

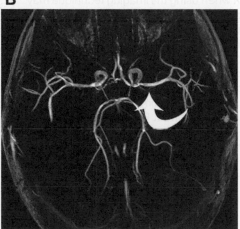

Fig. 11. Vasospasm. Status of a 4-year-old child post subarachnoid hemorrhage with altered mental status 1 week later. (*A*) Transtemporal Doppler of the MCA demonstrates markedly (increased peak systolic velocity (PSV) measuring 337 cm/s). (*B*) MRA confirmed the presence of narrowing of the left MCA (*arrow*), intracranial portions of the internal carotid arteries, left ACA, and basilar artery secondary to vasospasm.

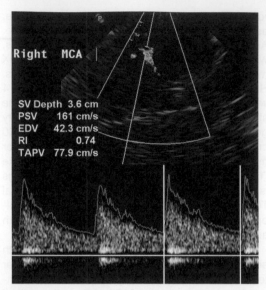

Right MCA

SV Depth 3.6 cm
PSV   161 cm/s
EDV   42.3 cm/s
RI   0.74
TAPV   77.9 cm/s

Fig. 12. Twelve-year-old boy with headaches. Transtemporal tracing of the MCA demonstrates increased RI suggestive of a common migraine.

significant difference in TAMMX measurements.[26,27] The reasons for these differing results are likely multifactorial. Centers should be aware of these potential differences when performing the STOP protocol and consider performing their own comparison studies when using imaging equipment. It is important to optimize instrument settings (volume size, gain, waveform display), and perform careful examinations so that the highest mean velocity is documented. With closer attention to technique, differences between the velocity data acquired with different ultrasound machines can be reduced. A 10% lower cut point for TAMMX when using the imaging technique may be appropriate depending on the protocol and machine used.[13] Jones and colleagues[13,96] reviewed the STOP data and reported that a PSV with velocities greater than 250 cm/s may be another useful value when assessing stroke risk in patients with sickle cell disease (**Fig. 13**). Although angle correction with TCDI may be a potential way to correct for lower velocities obtained by TCDI compared with nonimaging TCD, this technique has not yet been validated in a large

series and carries the risk of overestimating stroke risk in children with sickle cell disease.[29]

The STOP velocity criteria apply only to children with sickle cell anemia who have not had a previous stroke. Children with conditional velocities should be rescreened within 3 to 6 months, although those with normal studies may be rescreened yearly.[93] Increased ACA of 170 cm/s or higher, although not part of the STOP criteria, can also suggest an increased stroke risk.[99]

Optimal management for children with abnormal velocities remains problematic, with no consensus regarding long-term management in children with persistently abnormal velocities (**Fig. 14**). The side effects of prolonged transfusion therapy have clinicians searching for other methods of improving stroke risk, including the use of hydroxycarbamide (hydroxyurea) therapy and bone marrow transplant.[89,100–105] Although many children with conditional velocities remain in the conditional range for years or eventually normalize, up to 23% of this cohort eventually convert to abnormal.[100,101] Protocols using hydroxycarbamide (hydroxyurea) therapy in children with conditional velocities show promise and suggest that following these patients with TCD may be useful to assess treatment response.[103–105]

Intraoperative monitoring

Intraoperative TCD monitoring of MCA velocities during carotid endarterectomy is often performed in adults.[106] Intraoperative complications include ischemia during cross-clamping, hyperemic phenomena, or embolization of plaque. Hyperemic phenomena secondary to ischemia are depicted by a sudden increase in flow velocity. Solid or gaseous microemboli can be documented by TCD as high-amplitude spikes with a "chirping" sound.[107] TCD can be used to assess the effect of carotid cross-clamping on the MCA in children and adults.

TCD has shown that asymptomatic microemboli enter the cerebral circulation in large numbers during "routine" carotid angiography and pediatric scoliosis surgery. High rates of microemboli may be related to the presence of right to left cardiac shunts.[108,109]

Table 2 STOP risk categories	
Normal	<170 cm/s TAMMX
Conditional	170–199 cm/s TAMMX
Abnormal	>200 cm/s TAMMX in the MCA or distal ICA, >250 cm/s PSV

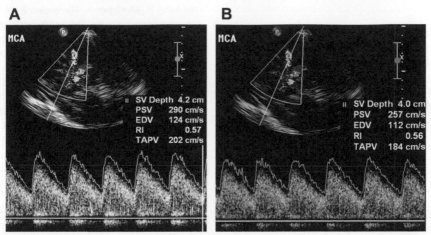

Fig. 13. Sickle cell disease: assessing risk of stroke using STOP criteria. (*A*) Transtemporal approach insonating the MCA demonstrates a PSV of 290 cm/s and TAMMX (TAPV) of 202 cm/s. These velocities are in the abnormal category for stroke risk. (*B*) Transtemporal approach insonating the MCA using the imaging technique demonstrates a PSV of 257 cm/s and TAMMX (TAPV) of 184 cm/s. Although TAMMX velocities are in the conditional range, this velocity may be slightly low due to the use of the imaging technique. The PSV of 257 cm/s suggests this patient is at high risk for stroke and close follow-up should be performed.

TCD monitoring during cardiopulmonary bypass for cardiac surgery is also being evaluated. TCD can demonstrate emboli showers that occur during aortic cannulation, cardiac manipulation, or other surgical maneuvers.[110–112] TCD has been used to monitor flow patterns during cardiopulmonary bypass, with a decrease in mean velocity with increasing hypothermia noted.[113] Hypothermic circulatory arrest and hypothermia with continuous low-flow cardiopulmonary bypass are used during the repair of complex congenital heart lesions. Extended periods of profound hypothermia may impair cerebral function and metabolism and can result in ischemic brain injury. TCD allows for noninvasive monitoring of cerebral perfusion during operations when circulatory arrest or low-flow bypass is being used. Monitoring may aid in the development of improved methods of cerebral protection during repair of complex congenital heart lesions.[108,113,114]

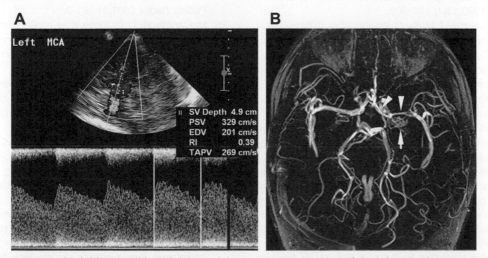

Fig. 14. Nine-year-old child with sickle cell disease. (*A*) Transtemporal tracing of the left MCA demonstrates markedly increased PSV measuring 329 cm/s and an abnormally increased TAMMX (TAPV) of 269 cm/s. (*B*) MRA confirms findings with narrowing of the left internal carotid artery and left MCA (*arrowheads*) and prominent left lenticulostriate branches (*arrow*) consistent with moyamoya disease.

SUMMARY

TCD can be used to evaluate cerebrovascular flow in many clinical circumstances. Information obtained may be useful in guiding therapy, but should be carefully correlated with clinical circumstances that are specific to each individual patient. Baseline and serial examinations are particularly useful if the TCD and clinical findings are unclear.

REFERENCES

1. Raju TNK. Cranial Doppler applications in neonatal critical care. Crit Care Clin 1992;8(1):93–111.
2. Saliba EM, Laugier J. Doppler assessment of the cerebral circulation in pediatric intensive care. Crit Care Clin 1992;8(1):79–92.
3. Taylor GA. Current concepts in neonatal cranial Doppler sonography. Ultrasound Q 1992;4:223–44.
4. Seibert JJ, McCowan TC, Chadduck WM, et al. Duplex pulsed Doppler US versus intracranial pressure in the neonate. Clinical and experimental studies. Radiology 1989;171:155–60.
5. Aeslid R. Transcranial Doppler sonography. J Neurosurg 1982;57:769–73.
6. Lupetin AR, Davis DA, Beckman I, et al. Transcranial Doppler sonography. Part 1. Principles, technique, and normal appearances. Radiographics 1995;15:179–87.
7. Katz ML, Comerota AJ. Transcranial Doppler: a review of technique, interpretation and clinical applications. Ultrasound Q 1991;8:241–9.
8. Byrd SM. An overview of transcranial Doppler color flow imaging: a technique comparison. Ultrasound Q 1996;13(4):197–202.
9. Rosendahl T, Muller C, Wagner W, et al. Transcranial imaging: a new angle on transcranial Doppler. Video J Color Flow Imaging 1995;5:60–2.
10. Fujioka KA, Douville CM. Anatomy and free hand examination techniques. In: Newell DW, Aaslid R, editors. Transcranial Doppler. New York: Raven Press; 1992. p. 9–31.
11. McCarville MB. Comparison of duplex and nonduplex transcranial Doppler ultrasonography. Ultrasound Q 2008;24:167–76.
12. Seibert JJ, Glasier CM, Leithiser RE Jr, et al. Transcranial Doppler using standard duplex equipment in children. Ultrasound Q 1990;8:167–75.
13. Bulas D. Screening children for sickle cell vasculopathy: guideline for transcranial Doppler evaluation. Pediatr Radiol 2005;35:235–41.
14. Rabe H, Grohs B, Schmidt RM, et al. Acoustic power measurements of Doppler ultrasound devices used for perinatal and infant examinations. Pediatr Radiol 1990;20:277–81.
15. Lizzi R, Mortimer A, Cartensen E, et al. Bioeffects considerations for the safety of diagnostic ultrasound. J Ultrasound Med 1988;7(Suppl):1–38.
16. Aaslid R. Transcranial Doppler sonography. New York: Springer-Verlag; 1986. p.10–21.
17. Archer LNJ, Evans DH, Levene MI. Doppler ultrasound examination of the anterior cerebral arteries of normal newborn infants. The effect of postnatal age. Early Hum Dev 1985;10:255–60.
18. Horgan JG, Rumack CM, Hay T, et al. Absolute intracranial blood-flow velocities evaluated by duplex Doppler sonography in asymptomatic preterm and term neonates. AJR Am J Roentgenol 1989;152:1059–64.
19. Allison JW, Faddis LA, Kinder DL, et al. Intracranial resistive index (RI) values in normal term infants during the first day of life. Pediatr Radiol 2000;30:618–20.
20. Chadduck WM, Seibert JJ. Intracranial duplex Doppler: practical uses in pediatric neurology and neurosurgery. J Child Neurol 1989;4(Suppl):S77–86.
21. Adams RJ, Nichols FT, McKie VC, et al. Transcranial Doppler: influence of hematocrit in children with sickle cell anemia without stroke. J Cardiovasc Tech 1989;8:97–101.
22. Adams RJ, Nichols FT III, Aaslid R, et al. Cerebral vessel stenosis in sickle cell disease: criteria for detection by transcranial Doppler. Am J Pediatr Hematol Oncol 1990;12:277–85.
23. Bulas DI, Jones A, Seibert J, et al. TCD screening for stroke prevention in sickle cell anemia (STOP): pitfalls in technique variation. Pediatr Radiol 2000;20:733–8.
24. Jones A, Seibert J, Nichols F, et al. Comparison of TCDI and TCD in children with sickle cell anemia. Pediatr Radiol 2001;31:461–9.
25. McCarville M, Li C, Xiong X, et al. Comparison of TCD sonography with and without imaging in the evaluation of children with sickle cell anemia. Am J Roentgenol 2003;183:1117–22.
26. Neish A, Blews D, Simms C, et al. Screening for stroke in sickle cell anemia: comparison of transcranial Doppler imaging and nonimaging US techniques. Radiology 2002;222:709–14.
27. Malouf AJ, Hamrick-Turner JE, Doherty MC, et al. Implementation of the STOP protocol for stroke prevention in sickle cell anemia by using duplex power Doppler imaging. Radiology 2001;219:359–65.
28. Fujioka KA, Gates DT, Spencer MP. A comparison of transcranial color Doppler imaging and standard static pulsed wave Doppler in the assessment of intracranial hemodynamics. J Vasc Tech 1994;18:29–35.
29. Krejza J, Rudzinski W, Pawlak MA, et al. Angle-corrected imaging transcranial Doppler sonography

versus imaging and nonimaging transcranial Doppler sonography in children with sickle cell disease. AJNR Am J Neuroradiol 2007;28:1613–8.

30. Winkler P, Helmke K. Major pitfalls in Doppler investigations with particular reference to the cerebral vascular system. Part I. Sources in error, resulting pitfalls, and measures to prevent errors. Pediatr Radiol 1990;20:219–28.

31. Winkler P, Helmke K, Mahl M. Major pitfalls in Doppler investigations. Part II. Low flow velocities and color Doppler applications. Pediatr Radiol 1990;20:304.

32. Dean LM, Taylor GA. The intracranial venous system in infants: normal and abnormal findings on duplex and color Doppler sonography. AJR Am J Roentgenol 1995;164:151–6.

33. Taylor GA. Intracranial venous system in the newborn: evaluation of normal anatomy and flow characteristics with color Doppler US. Radiology 1992;183:449–52.

34. Chen CY, Chou TY, Zimmerman RA, et al. Pericerebral fluid collection: differentiation of enlarged subarachnoid spaces from subdural collection with color Doppler US. Radiology 1996;201:389–92.

35. Tessler FN, Dion J, Vinuela F, et al. Cranial arteriovenous malformations in neonates: color Doppler imaging with angiographic correlation. AJR Am J Roentgenol 1989;153:1027–30.

36. Soto G, Daneman A, Hellman J. Doppler evaluation of cerebral arteries in a galenic vein malformation. J Ultrasound Med 1985;4:673–5.

37. Westra SJ, Curran JG, Duckwiler GR, et al. Pediatric intracranial vascular malformations: evaluation of treatment results with color Doppler US. Radiology 1993;186:775–83.

38. Lindegaard KF, Aaslid R, Nornes H. Cerebral arteriovenous malformations. In: Aaslid R, editor. Transcranial Doppler sonography. New York: Springer-Verlag; 1986. p. 86–105.

39. Lindegaard KF, Grolimund P, Aaslid R, et al. Evaluation of cerebral AVM's using transcranial Doppler ultrasound. J Neurosurg 1986;65:335–44.

40. Petty GW, Massaro AR, Tatemichi TK, et al. Transcranial Doppler ultrasonographic changes after treatment for AVMS. Stroke 1990;21:260–6.

41. Jordan LC, Wityk RJ, Dowling MM, et al. Transcranial Doppler ultrasound in children with Sturge Weber syndrome. J Child Neurol 2008;23(2): 137–43.

42. Duan YY, Xy Zhou, Liu X, et al. Carotid and transcranial color-coded duplex ultrasonography for the diagnosis of dural arteriovenous fistulas. Cerebrovasc Dis 2008;25(4):304–10.

43. Goh D, Minns RA. Intracranial pressure and cerebral arterial flow velocity indices in childhood hydrocephalus: current review. Childs Nerv Syst 1995;11:392–6.

44. Goh D, Minns RA, Hendry GMA, et al. Cerebrovascular resistive index assessed by duplex Doppler sonography and its relationship to intracranial pressure in infantile hydrocephalus. Pediatr Radiol 1992;22:246–50.

45. Klingelhofer J, Conrad B, Benecke R, et al. Evaluation of intracranial pressure from transcranial Doppler studies in cerebral disease. J Neurol 1988;235:159–62.

46. Bada HS, Miller JE, Menke JA, et al. Intracranial pressure and cerebral arterial pulsatile flow measurements in neonatal intraventricular hemorrhage. J Pediatr 1982;100:291–6.

47. Taylor GA, Phillips MD, Ichord RN, et al. Intracranial compliance in infants: evaluation with Doppler US. Radiology 1994;191:787–91.

48. Taylor GA, Madsen JR. Neonatal hydrocephalus: hemodynamic response to fontanelle compression: correlation with intracranial pressure and need for shunt placement. Radiology 1996;201: 685–9.

49. Westra SJ, Lazareff J, Curran JG, et al. Transcranial Doppler ultrasonography to evaluate need for cerebrospinal fluid drainage in hydrocephalic children. J Ultrasound Med 1998;17:561–9.

50. Westra SJ, Stotland MA, Lazareff J, et al. Perioperative transcranial Doppler US to evaluate intracranial compliance in young children undergoing craniosynostosis repair surgery. Radiology 2001; 218:816–23.

51. Hanlo PW, Gooskens RH, Nijhuis IJ, et al. Value of transcranial Doppler indices in predicting raised ICP in infantile hydrocephalus. Childs Nerv Syst 1995;11:595.

52. Rodriguez-Nunez A, Somoza-Martin M, Gomez-Lado C, et al. Therapeutic criteria in communicating childhood hydrocephalus. J Neurosurg Sci 2008;52(1):17–21.

53. Pople IK. Doppler flow velocities in children with controlled hydrocephalus: reference values for the diagnosis of blocked cerebrospinal fluid shunts. Childs Nerv Syst 1992;8(3):124–5.

54. Taylor GA, Trescher WH, Johnston MV, et al. Experimental neuronal injury in the newborn lamb: a comparison of N-methyl-D-aspartic acid receptor blockade and nitric oxide synthesis inhibition on lesion size and cerebral hyperemia. Pediatr Res 1995;38:644–51.

55. Blakenberg FG, Loh NN, Norbash AM, et al. Impaired cerebrovascular autoregulation after hypoxic-ischemic injury in extremely low-birth-weight neonates: detection with power and pulsed wave Doppler US. Radiology 1997;205(2):563–8.

56. Stark JE, Seibert JJ. Cerebral artery Doppler ultrasonography for prediction of outcome after perinatal asphyxia. J Ultrasound Med 1984;13: 595–600.

57. Gray PH, Tudehope DI, Massel JP, et al. Perinatal hypoxic-ischaemic brain injury: prediction of outcome. Dev Med Child Neurol 1993;35:965–73.

58. Archer LNJ, Levene ME, Evans DH. Cerebral artery Doppler ultrasonography for prediction of outcome after perinatal asphyxia. Lancet 1986;2:1116–8.

59. Raju TNK. Cerebral Doppler studies in the fetus and newborn infant. J Pediatr 1991;119(2):165–74.

60. Bellner J, Romner B, Reinstrup P, et al. Transcranial Doppler sonography pulsatility index (PI) reflects intracranial pressure. Surg Neurol 2004;62(1):45–51.

61. Bode H. Pediatric applications of transcranial Doppler sonography. New York: Springer-Verlag; 1988. p. 44–75.

62. Newell DW, Seiler RW, Aaslid R. Head injury and cerebral circulatory arrest. In: Newell DW, Aaslid R, editors. Transcranial Doppler. New York: Raven Press; 1992. p. 109–21.

63. Kirkham F, Levin S, Padayachee TS, et al. Transcranial pulsed Doppler ultrasound findings in brain stem death. J Neurol Neurosurg Psychiatry 1987;50:1504–13.

64. Powers AD, Graeber MC, Smith RR. Transcranial Doppler ultrasonography in the determination of brain death. Neurosurgery 1989;24:884–9.

65. Valentin A, Karuik R, Winkler WB, et al. Transcranial Doppler for early identification of potential organ transplant donors. Wien Klin Wochenschr 1997;109:837–9.

66. Petty GW, Wiebers DO, Meissner I. Transcranial Doppler ultrasonography: clinical applications in cerebrovascular disease. Mayo Clin Proc 1990;65:1350–64.

67. Chui NC, Shen EY, Lee BS. Reversal of diastolic cerebral blood flow in infants without brain death. Pediatr Neurol 1994;11:337–40.

68. Ducrocq X, Hassler W, Moritade K, et al. Consensus opinion on diagnosis of cerebral circulatory arrest using Doppler-sonography: Task Force Group on cerebral death of the Neurosonology Research Group of the World Federation of Neurology. J Neurol Sci 1998;159:145–50.

69. Glasier CM, Seibert JJ, Chadduck WM, et al. Brain death in infants: evaluation with Doppler US. Radiology 1989;172:377–80.

70. Shiogai T, Sato E, Tokitsu M, et al. Transcranial Doppler monitoring in severe brain damage: Relationships between intracranial haemodynamics, brain dysfunction, and outcome. Neurol Res 1990;12:205–13.

71. Feri M, Ralli L, Felici M, et al. Transcranial Doppler and brain death diagnosis. Crit Care Med 1994;22(7):1120–6.

72. Qian SY, Fan XM, Yin HH. Transcranial Doppler assessment of brain death in children. Singapore Med J 1998;39:247–50.

73. Hassler W, Steinmetz H, Gawlowski J. Transcranial Doppler ultrasonography in raised intracranial pressure and in intracranial circulatory arrest. J Neurosurg 1998;68:745–51.

74. Jalili M, Crade M, Davis AL. Carotid blood-flow velocity changes detected by Doppler ultrasound in determination of brain death in children: a preliminary report. Clin Pediatr 1994;33:669–74.

75. Wang K, Yuan Y, Xu ZQ, et al. Benefits of combination of electroencephalography, short latency somatosensory evoked potentials, and transcranial Doppler techniques for confirming brain death. J Zhejiang Univ Sci B 2008;9(11):916–20.

76. Lennihan L, Petty GW, Mohr JP, et al. Transcranial Doppler detection of anterior cerebral artery vasospasm [abstract]. Stroke 1989;20:151.

77. Sloan MA, Haley EC Jr, Kassell NF, et al. Sensitivity and specificity of transcranial Doppler ultrasonography in the diagnosis of vasospasm following subarachnoid hemorrhage. Neurology 1989;39:1514–8.

78. Kincaid MS. Transcranial Doppler ultrasonography: a diagnostic tool of increasing utility. Curr Opin Anaesthesiol 2008;21(5):552–9.

79. Rigamonti A, Ackery A, Baker AJ. Transcranial Doppler monitoring in subarachnoid hemorrhage: a critical tool in critical care. Can J Anaesth 2008;55(2):112–23.

80. Topeuoglu MA, Pryor JC, Oglvy CS, et al. Cerebral vasospasm following subarachnoid hemorrhage. Curr Treat Options Cardiovasc Med 2002;4(5):373–84.

81. Lysakowski C, Walder B, Costanza MC, et al. Transcranial Doppler vs. angiography I patients with vasospasm due to a ruptured cerebral aneurysm: a systematic review. Stroke 2001;32:2292–8.

82. Kincaid MS, Souter MJ, Treggiari MM, et al. Accuracy of transcranial Doppler ultrasonography and single-photon emission computed tomography in the diagnosis of angiographically demonstrated cerebral vasospasm. J Neurosurg 2009;110:67–72.

83. Thie A, Fuhlendorf A, Spitzer K, et al. Transcranial Doppler evaluation of common and classic migraine. Part I. Ultrasonic features during the headache-free period. Headache 1990;30:201–8.

84. Thie A, Fuhlendorf A, Spitzer K, et al. Transcranial Doppler evaluation of common and classic migraine. Part II. Ultrasonic features during attacks. Headache 1990;30:209–15.

85. Wang HS, Huo MF, Huang SC, et al. Transcranial ultrasound diagnosis of intracranial lesions in children with headaches. Pediatr Neurol 2002;26:43–6.

86. Powers D, Wilson B, Imbus C, et al. The natural history of stroke in sickle cell disease. Am J Med 1978;65:461–71.

87. Huttenlocher PR, Moohr JW, Johns I, et al. Cerebral blood flow in sickle cell cerebrovascular disease. Pediatrics 1984;73:615–21.

88. Adams R, McKie V, Nichols F, et al. The use of transcranial ultrasonography to predict stroke in sickle cell disease. N Engl J Med 1992;326:605–10.

89. Waters MC, Patience M, Leisenring W, et al. Bone marrow transplantation for sickle cell disease. N Engl J Med 1986;335:369–76.

90. Adams RJ, Aaslid R, Gammal TE, et al. Detection of cerebral vasculopathy in sickle cell disease using transcranial Doppler ultrasonography and magnetic resonance imaging: case report. Stroke 1988;19:518–20.

91. Adams RJ, Nichols FT, Figueroa R, et al. Transcranial Doppler correlation with cerebral angiography in sickle cell disease. Stroke 1992;23: 1073–7.

92. Seibert JJ, Miller SF, Kirby RS, et al. Cerebrovascular disease in symptomatic and asymptomatic patients with sickle cell anemia: screening with duplex transcranial Doppler US—correlation with MR imaging and MR angiography. Radiology 1993;189:457–66.

93. Nichols FT, Jones AM, Adams RJ, et al. Stroke prevention in sickle cell disease (STOP) study guidelines for transcranial Doppler testing. J Neuroimaging 2001;11:353–62.

94. Adams R, McKie VC, Hsu L, et al. Prevention of a first stroke by transfusions in children with sickle cell anemia and abnormal results on transcranial Doppler ultrasonography. N Engl J Med 1998; 339:5–11.

95. Adams R, McKie VC, Brambilla D, et al. Stroke prevention trial in sickle cell anemia: study design. Control Clin Trials 1998;19:110–29.

96. Jones A, Granger S, Brambilla D, et al. Can peak systolic be used for prediction of stroke in sickle cell anemia? Pediatr Radiol 2005;35(1):66 72.

97. Pegelow CH, Wang W, Granger S, et al. Silent infarcts in children with sickle cell anemia and abnormal cerebral artery velocity. Arch Neurol 2001;58:2017–21.

98. Wang WC, Gallagher DM, Pegelow CH, et al. A multi-center comparison of MRI and TCD in the evaluation of the central nervous system in children with sickle cell disease. Am J Pediatr Hematol Oncol 2000;22:335–9.

99. Kwiatkowski J, Granger S, Brambilla D, et al. Elevated blood flow velocity in the anterior cerebral artery and stroke risk in sickle cell disease: extended analysis from the STOP trial. Br J Haematol 2006;134:333–9.

100. Hankins J, Fortner G, McCarville B, et al. The natural history of conditional TCD flow velocities in children with sickle cell anaemia. Br J Haematol 2008;142:94–9.

101. Adams RJ, Brambilla DG, Grander S, et al. Stroke and conversion to high risk in children screened with TCD during the STOP study. Blood 2004;103: 3689–94.

102. McCarville M, Goodin G, Fortner G, et al. Evaluation of a comprehensive transcranial Doppler screening program for children with sickle cell anemia. Pediatr Blood Cancer 2008;50:818–21.

103. Bernaudin F, Verlhac S, Coic L, et al. Long term follow-up of pediatric sickle cell disease patients with abnormal high velocities on transcranial Doppler. Pediatr Radiol 2005;35(3):242–8.

104. Zimmerman S, Schultz W, Buergett S, et al. Hydroxyurea therapy lowers TCD flow velocities in children with sickle cell anemia. Blood 2007;110: 1043–7.

105. Kratovil T, Bulas D, Driscoll M, et al. Hydroxyurea therapy lowers TCD velocities in children with sickle cell disease. Pediatr Blood Cancer 2004; 47:894–900.

106. Lupetin AR, Davis DA, Beckman I, et al. Transcranial Doppler sonography. Part II. Evaluation of intracranial and extracranial abnormalities and procedural monitoring. Radiographics 1995;15: 193–209.

107. Albin MS, Bunegin BS, Garcia C, et al. Transcranial Doppler can image microaggregates of intracranial air and particulate matter. J Neurosurg Anesthesiol 1989;1:134–5.

108. Abdul-Khaliq H, Uhlig R, Bottcher W, et al. Factors influencing the change in cerebral hemodynamics in pediatric patients during and after corrective cardiac surgery of congenital heart diseases by means of full flow cardiopulmonary bypass. Perfusion 2002;17:179–85.

109. Rodriguez RA, Letts M, Jarvis J, et al. Cerebral microembolization during pediatric scoliosis surgery: a transcranial Doppler study. J Pediatr Orthop 2001;21:532–6.

110. Pugsley W. The use of Doppler ultrasound in the assessment of microemboli during cardiac surgery. Perfusion 1986;4:115–22.

111. Jordan WD, Voellinger DC, Doblar DD, et al. Microemboli detected by TCD monitoring in patients during carotid endarterectomy. Cardiovasc Surg 1999;7:33–8.

112. Dagirmanjian A, Davis DA, Rothful WE, et al. Silent cerebral microemboli occurring during carotid angiography: frequency as determined with Doppler sonography. AJR Am J Roentgenol 1993; 161:1037–40.

113. Burrows FA. Transcranial Doppler monitoring of cerebral perfusion during cardiopulmonary bypass. Ann Thorac Surg 1999;56(3):1482–4.

114. Williams GD, Ramamoorthy C. Brain monitoring and protection during pediatric cardiac surgery. Semin Cardiothorac Vasc Anesth 2007;11:23–33.

Ultrasound Imaging of the Neck in Children

Nancy R. Fefferman, MD*, Sarah Sarvis Milla, MD

KEYWORDS

- Ultrasound • Neck • Children • Thyroid • Neck masses

Lesions involving the pediatric neck are common and may involve any of the soft tissue, vascular, or osseous structures contained within this space. Imaging evaluation of the neck in children can be challenging. Although the cross-sectional imaging modalities of computed tomography (CT) and magnetic resonance imaging (MRI) provide excellent spatial resolution and superior tissue contrast, respectively, the inherent limitations in children are well known. These limitations include concerns regarding the radiation dose associated with CT and its potential carcinogenic effects. In addition, the relatively long examination time for MRI often requires sedation of younger pediatric patients. Ultrasound provides a relatively risk-free, rapid, noninvasive imaging modality that is particularly useful in children. Ultrasound has been accepted as an effective means of imaging the neck in children for a variety of indications, including the initial evaluation of palpable masses and conditions affecting the thyroid gland. The continuous technological advances in ultrasound equipment have led to improved resolution and increased utility of this imaging modality for characterization of pathologic processes involving the neck in children.

TECHNIQUE

The superficial nature of the structures in the small pediatric neck enables use of high-frequency (10 MHz and higher) linear array transducers for optimal imaging. Because linear array transducers may be too large for the smaller infant neck, the recently introduced high-frequency linear array small parts transducers with a very small footprint may be better suited for these cases. A 7.5-MHz linear array transducer may be required for improved resolution of deeper structures in the older child. A curved or sector transducer (6–8 MHz) often serves as an adjunct in assessing thyroid measurements in the older child. Grayscale images are typically acquired in the sagittal, transverse, and oblique planes to best demonstrate any palpable abnormality. Traditional sagittal and transverse gray-scale images of the thyroid gland are routinely acquired.

The child ideally should be in the supine position with the neck slightly hyperextended to optimize the field of view. Placing a rolled small towel behind the neck for support also helps to facilitate the image acquisition.

Color Doppler imaging and spectral tracings provide important information regarding vascular flow, which is helpful in the characterization of neck masses as well as abnormalities of the thyroid gland. The introduction of elastography and other technological advances on the horizon will likely be applicable to pediatric neck ultrasound in the near future, enabling improved utility of this imaging modality.

BENIGN NECK MASSES
Congenital Abnormalities

Cervical thymus

The thymus develops from the third and fourth pharyngeal pouches, and normally descends caudally and medially from the angle of the mandible to its definitive location in the anterior superior mediastinum. This descent occurs during early gestation between the sixth and tenth weeks.[1] Interruption of this normal thymic migration can result in thymic tissue abnormally positioned anywhere along the expected path of

Division of Pediatric Radiology, Department of Radiology, New York University Langone Medical Center, 560 First Avenue, RIRM 234, New York, NY 10016, USA
* Corresponding author.
E-mail address: nancy.fefferman@nyumc.org (N.R. Fefferman).

Ultrasound Clin 4 (2009) 553–569
doi:10.1016/j.cult.2009.10.001
1556-858X/09/$ – see front matter © 2009 Elsevier Inc. All rights reserved.

descent, most commonly in the lateral neck or suprasternal region.[2] This abnormality has been described as aberrant or ectopic cervical thymic tissue, which may present as an asymptomatic palpable soft tissue mass or as an incidental finding on neck ultrasound.[3–5] The aberrant thymus can present as a bulging mass in the suprasternal region exaggerated by increased intrathoracic pressure during Valsalva maneuver or crying. In addition, superior herniation of normally positioned mediastinal thymus can occur, presenting as an anterior cervical mass that appears with increased intrathoracic pressure.[6]

Familiarity with the ultrasound appearance of the normal thymus gland is useful in recognizing abnormally positioned normal thymic tissue and preventing unnecessary biopsy or resection. The sonographic characteristics of the normal thymus located both in the mediastinum and ectopically in the cervical region have been well described.[7–10] Sonographic appearance of thymic tissue is described as a well-circumscribed, homogeneous, hypoechoic mass with echogenic branching linear structures and multiple echogenic foci, representing connective tissue septa and blood vessels within the septa (**Fig. 1**).

The aberrant thymic tissue typically does not exert mass effect on the adjacent structures. However, cervical extension of mediastinal thymus has been described in association with the rare innominate artery or brachiocephalic trunk syndrome.[11] Even less common than aberrant thymic tissue is the cervical thymic cyst, which can present as a neck mass. Cervical thymic cysts are believed to occur as a result of cystic degeneration of Hassell corpuscles or cystic change within remnants of the thymopharyngeal duct.[12,13] These cysts may be unilocular or multilocular, and may contain clear fluid or blood.

Thyroglossal duct cyst

The thyroglossal duct cyst accounts for approximately 70% of all congenital cysts in the neck, and represents one of the most common congenital neck masses in children. In embryological terms the developing thyroid gland descends in the neck from the foramen cecum to assume its final position in the lower neck anterior to the second and third tracheal rings. The thyroglossal duct normally involutes by the eighth gestational week. Persistence of the thyroglossal duct or its remnants can give rise to cyst formation located anywhere along the path of the thyroid descent from the base of the tongue to the thyroid isthmus. Sixty-five percent of these cysts are located in the infrahyoid region, 20% are suprahyoid, and 15% are at the level of the hyoid bone. These cysts most commonly present during early childhood as an asymptomatic midline, or slightly off midline, palpable mass. However, they may be painful if complicated by infection. When the cyst is parasagittal in location, it is more commonly found slightly to the left of midline.[14]

The sonographic characteristics of thyroglossal duct cysts have been studied by several groups who report a spectrum of findings.[15–17] Uncomplicated thyroglossal duct cysts tend to be unilocular, well-margined, fairly thin-walled masses with a range of echotextures including anechoic, hypoechoic, and complex heterogeneous echo patterns, which have been described as a pseudosolid appearance (**Fig. 2**). Posterior acoustic

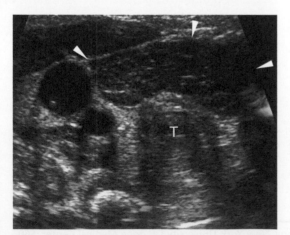

Fig. 1. Cervical thymus. Transverse ultrasound image of the lower cervical area shows a well-defined hypoechoic mass (*arrowheads*) anterior to the trachea (T) just inferior to the thyroid with internal echogenic foci and branching linear structures.

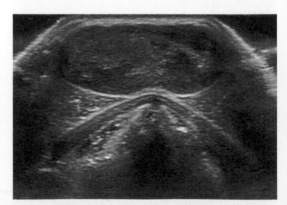

Fig. 2. Thyroglossal duct cyst. Midline transverse ultrasound of the infrahyoid region in a 2-year-old with a palpable mass demonstrates a well-circumscribed complex cystic mass embedded in the strap muscles.

enhancement is associated with the anechoic and hypoechoic lesions. However, this may be subtle or difficult to appreciate with the more complex lesions. The internal echotexture reflects the composition of the cystic contents, specifically the proteinaceous fluid secreted by the epithelial lining. Thyroglossal duct cysts complicated by inflammation may demonstrate a thickened, irregular wall with internal septa. Color Doppler interrogation often shows increased flow within the wall of the cyst and in the adjacent soft tissues when they are infected or inflamed (**Fig. 3**).

In rare cases, ectopic thyroid tissue may be present within the thyroglossal duct cyst, reported to occur in 0.5% to 5.7%.[18,19] Sonographic demonstration of the normal thyroid gland is necessary prior surgical resection of the thyroglossal duct cyst (Sistrunk procedure) to prevent potential resection of the patient's only functioning thyroid tissue.[20]

Dermoid and epidermoid inclusion cyst and teratoma

Included in the differential diagnosis of midline neck masses in children are dermoid and epidermoid inclusion cysts, which share a common origin. These cysts result from the trapping of ectoderm and mesoderm during midline fusion. The epidermoid is an ectodermally derived inclusion cyst lined by squamous cells, and contains proteinaceous debris, predominantly keratin. The dermoid is similar to the epidermoid but contains mesodermal derivatives including hair, sebaceous glands, and sweat glands. These cysts can be difficult to distinguish from thyroglossal duct cysts on physical as well as on sonographic evaluation.

Dermoid cysts tend to be suprahyoid in location in contrast to the thyroglossal duct cysts, which are more commonly infrahyoid. The epidermoid inclusion cyst may be more lateral in location. The more common sonographic features include a well-circumscribed echogenic mass. However, cysts showing a more hypoechoic echotexture have also been described (**Fig. 4**). Dermoid cysts may demonstrate a more heterogeneous echotexture, depending on the internal contents of the cyst.[21]

Teratomas are germ-cell tumors comprising all 3 germ-cell layers. Approximately 7% to 9% of teratomas occur in the head and neck region. Cervical teratomas are rare neck masses that are usually present at birth. Although these tumors are usually benign, malignant transformation can occur. These masses tend to be large, multiloculated, complex cystic lesions. The echotexture reflects the tumoral contents, which include fat, teeth, and soft tissue elements.[22,23]

Branchial cleft cysts

Neck masses in children may also be related to developmental anomalies of the branchial apparatus, the anlagen of the mature structures of the head and neck. The branchial apparatus consists of 6 branchial arches separated by 5 branchial clefts. Branchial apparatus anomalies include sinus tract, fistulous tract, and most commonly cyst formation, which are believed to occur as a result of incomplete regression of the branchial clefts and arches. Branchial cleft cysts represent the most common noninflammatory lateral neck masses in children and the second most common congenital neck lesions in children after the

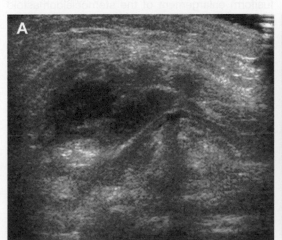
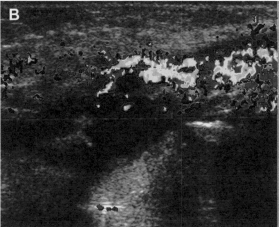

Fig. 3. Infected thyroglossal duct cyst. (*A*) Midline transverse ultrasound image of the infrahyoid region shows a complex cystic structure to the right of midline with marked thickening of the adjacent soft tissues. (*B*) Color Doppler image shows significant surrounding soft tissue hyperemia.

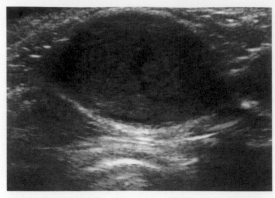

Fig. 4. Epidermoid inclusion cyst. Transverse image of the suprahyoid neck in a 5-year-old with a palpable neck mass shows a well-circumscribed hypoechoic mass with posterior acoustic enhancement containing low-level internal echoes.

thyroglossal duct cyst. The branchial cleft anomalies are generally classified as first, second, third, and fourth arch anomalies depending on the cleft or pouch of origin, with approximately 90% arising from the second branchial cleft and 8% from the first branchial cleft. Anomalies of the third and fourth branchial clefts are extremely rare.[24,25]

The location of the branchial cleft cysts parallels the embryologic development of the branchial arches into their normal anatomic structures. The first branchial cleft anomalies are closely associated with the parotid gland near the lower pole. Although the second branchial cleft anomalies can be found anywhere along the path of development of the second branchial cleft complex, they are most commonly found anterior to the sternocleidomastoid muscle in the anterior cervical triangle near the angle of the mandible.[26] The classic clinical presentation of branchial cleft cysts includes a recurrent, nontender, soft mass in the neck. These cysts may become enlarged and painful when complicated by infection or hemorrhage. Sonographic evaluation demonstrates a variable appearance, ranging from a thin-walled, discrete anechoic mass with posterior acoustic enhancement typical for cystic structures to a more complex cystic mass. Occasionally the branchial cleft cysts may contain cholesterol crystals resulting in debris. In the setting of infection or hemorrhage, the cyst wall may become thickened and irregular with increasing heterogeneity of the echotexture.[27]

Fibromatois colli

Fibromatosis colli, also known as sternocleidomastoid tumor of infancy due to its masslike enlargement of the sternocleidomastoid muscle,

is a benign pathologic process affecting the sternocleidomastoid muscle in neonates and young infants. This lesion typically manifests clinically approximately 2 weeks after birth as a palpable, nontender, firm, lateral neck mass in a baby presenting with torticollis. A clinical history of breech presentation or difficult delivery can usually be elicited in association with the physical findings. The mass histologically comprises collagen fibers and fibroblasts surrounding atrophied muscle fibers.[28] This configuration supports the current hypothesis for the pathophysiology of fibromatosis colli suggesting that occlusion of venous outflow from the sternocleidomastoid muscle during manipulation of the neck at delivery results in injury to muscle fibers and subsequent fibrosis.[29] This proposal has replaced the previous hypothesis that fibromatosis colli represented a hematoma within the sternocleidomastoid muscle.

Imaging findings of fibromatosis colli have been well described for ultrasound, CT, and MRI.[30–32] However, the characteristic sonographic findings of fibromatosis colli are usually diagnostic, making this the modality of choice in the imaging evaluation, reserving the more advanced cross-sectional imaging techniques of CT and MRI as problem-solving modalities when the clinical presentation or sonographic findings are atypical. The differential diagnosis includes the cadre of benign and malignant soft tissue masses of the neck in children, most commonly lymphoma, rhabdomyosarcoma, neuroblastoma, and lymphadenitis.

The classic ultrasound appearance of fibromatosis colli demonstrates a focal hyperechoic mass localized within the body of the sternocleidomastoid muscle (**Fig. 5**A). Alternatively fibromatosis colli may present sonographically as diffuse fusiform enlargement of the sternocleidomastoid muscle with a heterogeneous echotexture more commonly hyperechoic, reflecting disruption of the normal striated muscle pattern (**Fig. 5**B).[33] This appearance is often best appreciated by comparison with the size and echotexture of the contralateral unaffected sternocleidomastoid muscle in the sagittal and transverse planes (**Fig. 5**C). The normal echotexture of the striated sternocleidomastoid muscle compressed by the focal or diffuse mass may be identified adjacent to the mass at the periphery. Variable sonographic appearances of fibromatosis colli have also been reported, including the presence of 2 focal echogenic masses reflecting involvement of both the sternal and clavicular heads of the sternocleidomastoid muscle[33]; this is most apparent on the transverse images (**Fig. 5**D). Calcifications within the mass presenting as echogenic foci have been reported, but are quite rare.[29] Color Doppler

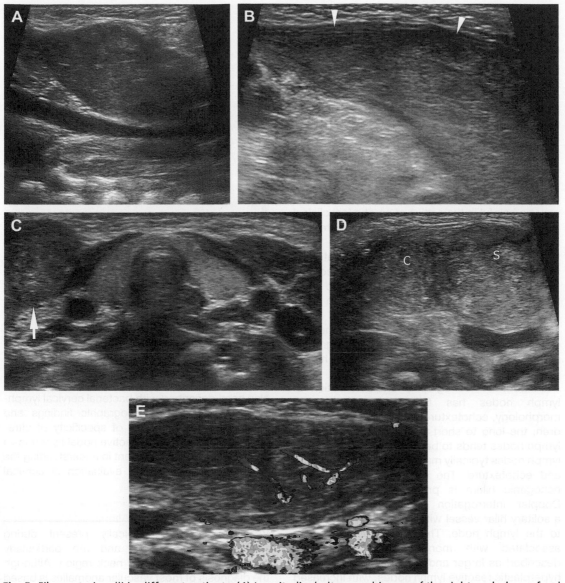

Fig. 5. Fibromatosis colli in different patients. (*A*) Longitudinal ultrasound image of the right neck shows focal enlargement of the sternocleidomastoid muscle with a heterogeneous echogenic mass and loss of the normal striated muscle echotexture. (*B*) Longitudinal ultrasound image of the right neck shows fusiform enlargement of the right sternocleidomastoid muscle. The compressed normal muscle fibers can be seen in the periphery (*arrowheads*). (*C*) Transverse ultrasound of the neck at the level of the thyroid gland showing asymmetric enlargement of the right sternocleidomastoid muscle (*arrow*). (*D*) Transverse ultrasound image of the right neck shows focal echogenic masses in the sternal (*S*) and clavicular (*C*) heads of the right sternocleidomastoid muscle. (*E*) Longitudinal color Doppler ultrasound image of the left neck demonstrates diffuse enlargement of the left sternocleidomastoid muscle with hyperemia.

interrogation can demonstrate hyperemia within the mass (**Fig. 5**E). Because fibromatosis colli and the associated torticollis usually resolve spontaneously, it is not surprising that the sonographic findings will vary depending on the temporal relationship of the imaging to the natural history of this process.

Infection

Cervical lymphadenopathy and lymphadenitis
Enlarged cervical lymph nodes are a frequent finding in children, and may present as a palpable neck mass. Reactive hyperplasia and infection are the most common causes for cervical lymphadenopathy in children. However, neoplastic

processes and underlying systemic diseases can also cause cervical lymphadenopathy and should be considered in the differential diagnosis. Reactive lymph node hyperplasia is usually transient and self-limited in response to a local or systemic infection. Cervical lymphadenitis is also a relatively common disease process affecting children, and is usually viral or bacterial in origin. The concentration of lymph nodes in the neck and the frequency of oropharyngeal infections in children contribute to the frequency of cervical lymphadenitis in children.[34,35] The typical clinical presentation includes nodal enlargement, erythema, and swelling of the overlying skin. Imaging evaluation with ultrasound may be helpful in the setting of an atypical clinical presentation, persistent symptoms refractory to antibiotic therapy, or recurrent symptoms. Ultrasound is often included in the initial evaluation of suspected cervical lymphadenopathy to confirm the diagnosis, because congenital cystic neck lesions can mimic enlarged lymph nodes on physical examination.

Although the specificity of ultrasound for cervical lymphadenopathy is limited, sonographic features of reactive cervical lymph node hyperplasia and cervical lymphadenitis have been described.[36,37] Sonographic characterization of lymph nodes has focused on the size, morphology, echotexture, and vascularity. In children, the long to short axis ratio of hyperplastic lymph nodes tends to be greater than 2. Reactive lymph nodes typically maintain their general shape and echotexture. The distinct oval shape and echogenic hilum is preserved (**Fig. 6**). Color Doppler interrogation generally demonstrates a solitary hilar vessel with a radial pattern of flow to the lymph node. The reactive lymph nodes associated with mononucleosis have been described as larger and rounder than the typical hyperplastic reactive lymph nodes, with increased vascularity.[37] The enlarged lymph nodes due to cervical lymphadenitis have been reported to have a long to short axis ratio tending to be less than 2. These infected lymph nodes may present as a nodal mass or phlegmon, with indistinct margins or a multilocular complex collection. The normal echogenic hilum is often distorted by the central inflammatory changes, with a residual narrow hilum of heterogeneous echotexture or even absence of the hilum (**Fig. 7**). Central hypoechoic or anechoic areas become more apparent in suppurative lymphadenitis as necrosis progresses and abscess formation ensues. Absence of central blood flow on color Doppler has been shown to be a good indicator for the presence of an abscess.[38] However, this may be difficult to accurately assess in the acutely ill, uncooperative child. Color

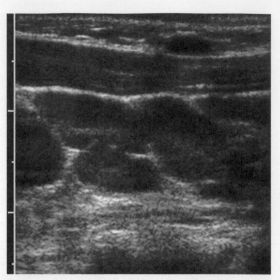

Fig. 6. Reactive cervical lymphadenopathy. Longitudinal ultrasound image of the left posterior neck shows a cluster of prominent cervical lymph nodes with an oval shape and central region of increased echogenicity.

Doppler interrogation may show an interrupted pattern of flow within the nodes or generalized avascularity. Peripheral increased vascularity has also been described with bacterial cervical lymphadenitis. Overlap of sonographic findings and subsequent inherent lack of specificity of ultrasound in distinguishing reactive nodal hyperplasia from malignancy is important in understanding the role of ultrasound in the evaluation of cervical lymphadenopathy.[39]

Vascular Anomalies

Vascular anomalies typically present during infancy and childhood, and are particularly common in the head and neck region. Although the diagnosis of most vascular anomalies is based on clinical history and physical examination, imaging is often used for confirmation of the suspected diagnosis, evaluation of extent of the lesion, pretreatment planning, and posttreatment monitoring.[40,41] Vascular anomalies can be divided into 2 major categories: hemangiomas and vascular malformations.[41] Hemangiomas are true, benign soft tissue tumors characterized by endothelial proliferation of capillary sized vessels. Typically diagnosed within the first 3 months of life, hemangiomas tend to proliferate within the first year of life, and regress in the following 1 to 5 years. Vascular malformations, in contradistinction, are congenital abnormalities of vascular or lymphatic formation, have normal endothelial turnover, and are formations of abnormal channels rather than a soft tissue mass. Although they

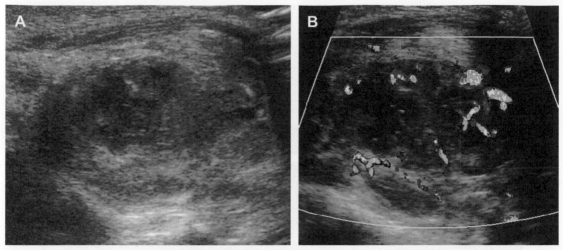

Fig. 7. Cervical lymphadenitis. (*A*) Longitudinal gray-scale and (*B*) color Doppler ultrasound images of the left posterior neck demonstrate a thick-walled, complex inflammatory mass with peripheral hyperemia.

may demonstrate evolution, particularly during hormonal changes associated with puberty, pregnancy, and hormone administration, they are not tumors. Vascular malformations are classified by the dominant channel type including capillary, arterial, venous and lymphatic, or combinations of channel type such as arteriovenous, venolymphatic, and capillary-lymphatic. Sonography for evaluation of hemangiomas and vascular malformations is often best performed with high-resolution linear array transducers. Low-flow color Doppler settings optimize visualization of the small vessels. High-sensitivity power Doppler with a low wall filter can also be used for the detection of the low-flow arterial and venous flow. Doppler interrogation and spectral waveform analysis of the intralesional vascularity is integral for the appropriate classification of vascular anomalies.

Hemangiomas

Hemangiomas, the most common vascular anomaly in the head and neck, are commonly diagnosed clinically as well-circumscribed, soft, red superficial masses. However, when these lesions are subcutaneous or located in the deep soft tissues, clinical diagnosis may be more difficult. Sonography is often the initial imaging study obtained in the evaluation of these suspected hemangiomas. The typical sonographic characterization of a hemangioma during the proliferative phase is a solid, well-circumscribed, soft tissue mass with increased vascularity, including both high-velocity arterial and low-resistance venous Doppler waveforms (**Fig. 8**).[42] Studies looking at gray-scale and Doppler characterization of hemangiomas have found that the presence of

a soft tissue mass is essential in distinguishing hemangiomas from other vascular anomalies.[42] In addition, color Doppler demonstration of high vessel density (>5 vessels per square centimeter) and a maximum Doppler shift exceeding 2 kHz are helpful in distinguishing hemangiomas from other infantile soft tissue masses.[43] It has been suggested, however, that current sonographic equipment may make the characterization of Doppler shift difficult and that velocity measurements may be underestimated due to lack of appropriate angle correction.[42] The presence of calcifications, ill-defined borders, or a poorly vascularized soft tissue mass should raise suspicion of malignancy, as these characteristics are associated with other rare infantile vascular soft tissue tumors.[44] In addition, an atypical clinical presentation for hemangioma should also prompt further investigation.

Vascular malformations

Vascular malformations are divided into low-flow and high-flow lesions, based on the character of the channels comprising the abnormality. Low-flow abnormalities include venous malformations, lymphatic malformations, capillary malformations, venolymphatic, and capillary-lymphatic malformations. Venous vascular malformations and lymphatic malformations are common in the head and neck region. Sonographic findings of venous malformations can include multiple hypoechoic channels in a sinusoidal or spongelike pattern that may contain low to intermediate echoes on gray-scale imaging, due to slow or stagnant flow.[42,45] Phleboliths have been described in 20% to 80% of venous vascular

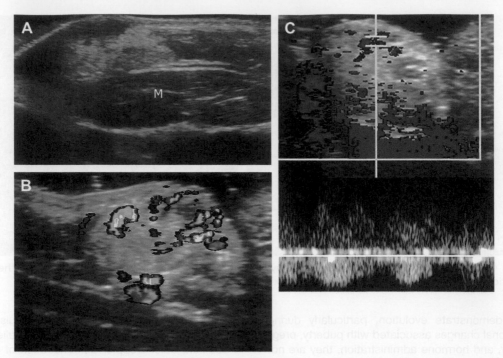

Fig. 8. Hemangioma. (*A*) Transverse sonogram of the right neck in a 3-month-old with discoloration of the skin demonstrates a predominantly hyperechoic mass superficial to underlying muscle (M) in the subcutaneous soft tissues of the neck. (*B*) Longitudinal color Doppler image shows significant vascularity within the mass. (*C*) Doppler interrogation of the internal vascularity demonstrates arterial waveforms.

malformations.[45,46] Phleboliths may be identified sonographically within the channels as mobile, hyperechoic, shadowing structures. Doppler imaging typically demonstrates monophasic low-velocity flow within these malformations. However, approximately 7% to 10% of venous vascular malformations may not demonstrate venous flow on Doppler interrogation.[42,45] As a result of the inherent slow flow, venous vascular malformations are susceptible to thrombosis, causing acute signs and symptoms of redness, swelling, and pain. This complication manifests sonographically with increased echogenicity within the venous sinusoids.

Lymphatic malformations are composed of both macrocystic and microcystic components. The typical sonographic gray-scale appearance includes multiple thin-walled cystic structures of varying sizes, reflecting the macrocystic components (**Fig. 9**). In addition, septations, echogenic material, and fluid/fluid levels due to hemorrhage may be identified within these macrocysts. On ultrasound, the microcystic components of lymphatic malformations appear as an echogenic mass due to the multiple interfaces created by the small cysts. The cystic spaces of lymphatic malformations are generally avascular on color

Doppler interrogation. The internal septations may demonstrate both arterial and venous flow, with reportedly higher resistive index values compared with hemangiomas and arteriovenous malformations, and relatively low mean venous peak velocities. However, the utility of these quantitative measures remains uncertain, as variation is noted.[42] Lymphatic malformations may become infected, causing the cystic structures to appear thick-walled with increased peripheral vascularity. Frequently large venous and lymphatic malformations may occupy more than one anatomic space within the neck, and thus may not be completely imaged by ultrasound; MRI is often a necessary adjunct in evaluation for treatment.

Arteriovenous malformations consist of multiple abnormal communications between arteries and veins on the capillary level. The classic gray-scale sonographic findings of arteriovenous malformations include multiple tortuous, hypoechoic channels in the absence of a soft tissue mass[42] (**Fig. 10**). These lesions demonstrate characteristic high-flow low resistance arterial and venous waveforms on Color Doppler interrogation.[42] Arterialization of draining veins can be seen.[47] After initial ultrasound evaluation, patients with arteriovenous malformations typically undergo further imaging

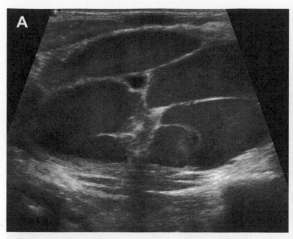
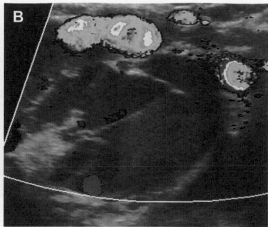

Fig. 9. Lymphatic malformation. (*A*) Longitudinal sonogram of the right neck in a 2-year-old with a chronic soft palpable abnormality of the neck demonstrates a multiloculated hypoechoic structure with linear septations, low-level echoes, and posterior acoustic enhancement. (*B*) Color Doppler imaging shows no vascular flow within the multilocular cystic collection, with minimal flow in the septations.

with CT angiography, MR angiography, or conventional angiography for assessment of potential treatment with embolization or surgery.

Capillary malformation such as port wine stains have not been shown to demonstrate significant sonographic findings. These lesions show either no sonographic findings or mild isoechoic thickening of the affected skin and subcutaneous tissues without obvious abnormal vascular flow.[42]

MALIGNANT SOFT TISSUE NECK MASSES

In the pediatric population, malignant soft tissue masses presenting in the neck are uncommon. Lymphoma, rhabdomyosarcoma, and neuroblastoma are common tumors in childhood, and are the most likely malignant tumors to present as a palpable neck mass. The sonographic findings of these individual soft tissue tumors in the location of the head and neck have not been particularly well described. However, the overall sonographic findings of malignant lymph nodes are well documented. Gray-scale sonographic findings suggesting nodal malignancy include abnormally increased size, change of shape, and abnormal internal architecture.[48] Malignant lymph nodes tend to have increased transverse dimension with loss of the more typical oblong configuration. In the absence of clinical signs and symptoms of lymphadenitis, the loss of normal hilar vessel/fat architecture and presence of intranodal necrosis are suggestive of a malignancy. Doppler sonography can detect abnormal lymph node vascularity including peripheral and nonhilar vascularity. Elevated lymph node vascular resistance has been suggested to denote malignant

involvement.[49] The presence of any of these findings should prompt biopsy. Ultrasound is an ideal modality for image-guided biopsy, and typically yields the accurate pathologic diagnosis.[50] In addition to ultrasound-guided biopsy, patients who are diagnosed with soft tissue malignancies will usually undergo further evaluation with CT or MRI, as well as possibly ^{18}F-fluorodeoxyglucose positron emission tomography for lymphoma, and ^{131}I-metaiodobenzylguanidine (MIBG) imaging for neuroblastoma, to assess extent of local and metastatic disease.

Lymphoma

Leukemia and lymphoma are the most common malignancies in childhood, and have also been described as the most common malignancies in the pediatric neck.[22] The characteristic sonographic findings of lymphomatous nodes include enlarged nodes with an isoechoic to hypoechoic echotexture with loss of the normal central hilar architecture.[36,51] Increased and abnormal nonhilar vascularity is described with Doppler imaging. Although these findings may be associated with lymphoma, they remain nonspecific and may overlap with lymphadenitis. However, these patients will not improve on antibiotics. Close follow-up is usually advised, and subsequent biopsy will render the appropriate diagnosis in those cases that do not resolve.

Rhabdomyosarcoma

Although rhabdomyosarcoma is a rare soft tissue neoplasm, 40% of cases are found in the head and neck, most commonly in the sinonasal region.

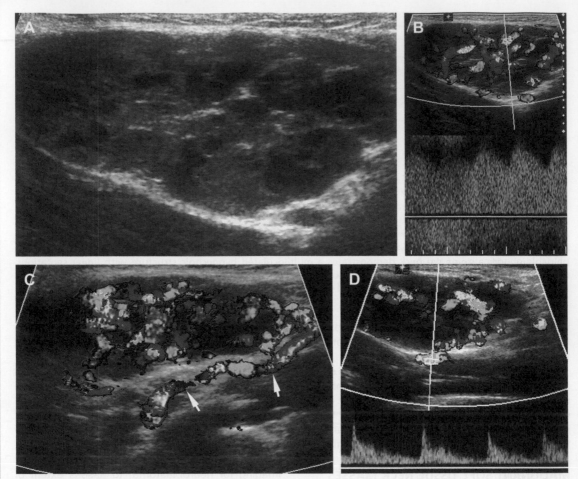

Fig. 10. Arteriovenous malformation. (*A*) Longitudinal gray-scale sonography of the left neck in a 5-year-old girl with a palpable neck mass shows a cluster of medium sized hypoechoic tubular structures. (*B*) Color Doppler evaluation confirms blood flow. Interrogation of the vessels shows high diastolic arterial flow and arterialization of venous waveforms. (*C*) Transverse imaging illustrates a prominent vessel (*arrows*) leading to the vascular channels. A few other prominent feeding vessels were also seen (not shown). (*D*) Doppler interrogation demonstrates another arterial feeding vessel.

Limited sonographic description exists for rhabdo-myosarcoma, because the more advanced cross-sectional imaging modalities of CT and MRI are usually obtained for evaluation of local and metastatic disease. However, the initial diagnosis may be suggested on ultrasound, which has been shown to demonstrate a well-defined, slightly hypoechoic inhomogeneous mass with significantly increased flow.[52]

Neuroblastoma

Although neuroblastoma is a relatively common malignancy affecting children, primary cervical neuroblastoma is rare, comprising less than 5% of all neuroblastoma cases. Cervical neuroblastoma often presents as a palpable neck mass associated with feeding and respiratory

difficulties. Sonographic characteristics of cervical neuroblastoma are relatively nonspecific, and include a hypoechoic mass with varying degrees of heterogeneity and vascularity. Calcifications may be present with shadowing echogenic foci (**Fig. 11**). Sonography may also demonstrate enlarged cervical lymph nodes.[50,53] Because ultrasound is nonspecific, further imaging with CT, MRI, and MIBG are usually necessary, in addition to biopsy.

THYROID ABNORMALITIES

Although thyroid disease is more common in the adult population, it does affect children, and ultrasound is an ideal modality for the initial imaging evaluation. The sonographic characteristics of the normal thyroid gland as well as the pathologic

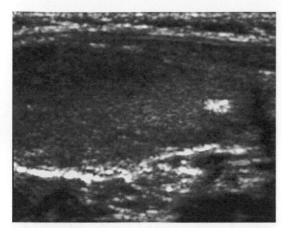

Fig. 11. Neuroblastoma. Transverse ultrasound image of the right neck shows a well-circumscribed hypoechoic mass with a single shadowing echogenic focus due to a calcification.

processes affecting the thyroid gland have been well described in the literature. Abnormalities of the thyroid gland include congenital thyroid disorders, benign and malignant masses, and diffuse thyroid diseases. The normal thyroid gland is a bilobed structure, which demonstrates a homogeneous echotexture that is moderately hyperechoic relative to the adjacent musculature. The size of the thyroid gland with respect to linear dimensions and volume is an important part of the sonographic evaluation, and normative values are available for comparison both in the literature and on-line.[54–57]

Congenital Thyroid Disorders

Congenital hypothyroidism

Congenital hypothyroidism is a difficult clinical diagnosis in the newborn period when it is most critical due to the absence of physical findings. Because delayed diagnosis results in the devastating consequences of irreversible mental retardation and delayed bone growth, neonatal screening has become a routine part of newborn health care. Congenital hypothyroidism is reported to occur in approximately one in 3000 to 4000 infants[58,59] with a female to male ratio of 2 to 1. Thyroid dysgenesis accounts for about 85% of the cases of congenital hypothyroidism, with two-thirds attributed to ectopic location of thyroid tissue due to incomplete or aberrant thyroid migration. Complete absence of the thyroid gland is significantly less common and accounts for approximately one-third of cases of thyroid dysgenesis. Dyshormonogenesis or functional thyroid glandular defects secondary to abnormalities in one or more of the enzymes necessary for

the synthesis and secretion of thyroid hormones comprise the remaining 10% to 20% of congenital hypothyroidism. In contrast to thyroid dysgenesis, which is more commonly sporadic, dyshormonogenesis is usually genetically transmitted.[14]

Ultrasound can play an important role in the initial imaging evaluation of congenital hypothyroidism to determine the etiology and to help guide management.[60] Sonographic demonstration of normal-appearing thyroid glandular tissue in the normal location in the setting of congenital hypothyroidism has been classified as eutopic, indicating the presence of a normal thyroid gland or dyshormonogenesis. Absence of thyroid glandular tissue in the normal expected location has been classified as noneutopic thyroid, suggesting dysgenesis encompassing complete absence of the thyroid, hypoplasia, and ectopic thyroid (Fig. 12).[60] However, the detection of ectopic thyroid glandular tissue, which can be located anywhere along the course of the thyroglossal duct from the base of the tongue, is limited with gray-scale sonography.[61] Color Doppler ultrasound has been shown to be more sensitive than gray-scale ultrasound in the identification of ectopic thyroid glandular tissue. Ohnishi and colleagues[62] demonstrated 2 patterns of vascularity associated with ectopic thyroid tissue around the tongue area, including a peripheral type vascular pattern and internal color signal within the region of ectopic thyroid. Ectopic thyroid glandular tissue may also be present within a thyroglossal duct cyst. In dyshormonogenesis, the thyroid gland often becomes diffusely enlarged with a normal echotexture (Fig. 13).[14]

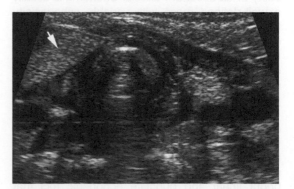

Fig. 12. Ectopic thyroid. Transverse midline sonographic image of the neck in a 2-week-old female with congenital hypothyroidism shows absence of the normal thyroid glandular tissue. A triangular soft tissue mass (arrow) with the echotexture of thyroid gland is present superior to the expected location of the thyroid.

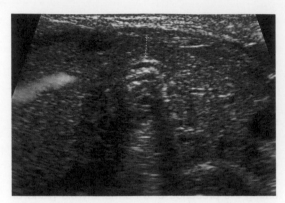

Fig. 13. Dyshormonogenesis. Transverse midline sonographic image of the thyroid in a newborn with congenital hypothyroidism demonstrates a diffusely enlarged thyroid gland with normal echotexture.

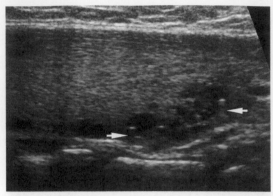

Fig. 14. Colloid cysts. Longitudinal sonographic image of the right lobe of the thyroid in a 12-year-old girl shows an ill-defined anechoic region in the inferior aspect of the lobe, with scattered punctate internal bright echogenic foci with associated comet tail artifacts (*arrows*).

Benign Thyroid Masses

Thyroid nodules are uncommon in the pediatric population, with a reported incidence on the order of 1%.[63,64] Approximately 85% of pediatric thyroid nodules are benign with the differential diagnosis, including follicular adenoma and cysts that usually represent degenerating nodules. Asymmetric enlargement of the thyroid gland in nodular hyperplasia or goiter may present clinically as a thyroid nodule. In addition, thyroid nodules can be found in association with diffuse thyroid diseases such as thyroiditis.[65]

Although the ultrasound characteristics associated with follicular adenoma have been described, the well-known overlap in the sonographic features of follicular carcinoma limit the diagnostic utility of ultrasound. Follicular adenoma is usually a well-defined mass with variable echogenicity that may be isoechoic, hyperechoic, or honeycomb in appearance. Presence of a peripheral thick, smooth hypoechoic halo has also been described, postulated to reflect the surrounding fibrous capsule or compressed adjacent thyroid parenchyma.[66]

Cysts or degenerating thyroid nodules may contain serous or colloid fluid or hemorrhage, with the sonographic appearance reflecting the internal contents. Colloid cysts are predominantly anechoic regions with scattered internal bright linear and punctate echogenic foci that may demonstrate associated comet tail artifact due to the presence of microcrystals (**Fig. 14**). Degenerating nodules may also demonstrate septations and calcifications. Peripheral hypervascularity is present on color Doppler interrogation.[66,67]

Malignant Thyroid Masses

Although the majority of thyroid nodules in the pediatric population are benign, there is a reported increased incidence of malignancy in the nodules found in children compared with adults.[68] Recent data suggest an incidence of malignancy of 16% in solitary thyroid nodules in children.[69] Thyroid carcinoma accounts for about 0.5% to 1.5% of all malignancies in children, with the incidence increasing from childhood to adolescence and in high-risk populations, including those exposed to high levels of ionizing radiation.[70,71] The clinical course of thyroid carcinoma in children has been shown to be different than in adults, with disease often presenting at a more advanced stage, larger size and increased incidence of lymph node involvement and lung metastasis. Thyroid carcinoma in children has been reported to have a better prognosis than thyroid carcinoma in adults despite a higher risk of recurrence.[72–74]

Similar to the adult population, papillary carcinoma is the most common form of thyroid cancer affecting children, accounting for approximately 80% of the cases. Papillary carcinoma spreads via the lymphatic system, resulting in early lymph node involvement (**Fig. 15**). Follicular carcinoma is the next most common pediatric thyroid malignancy, representing 17% of cases.[75] Medullary carcinoma accounts for approximately 2% to 3% of cases of thyroid malignancy in children, and is associated with multiple endocrine neoplasia types 2a and 2b.

Although sonographic characteristics have been described for thyroid malignancies, it is important to realize that ultrasound is limited in

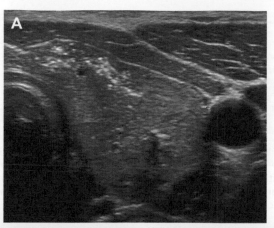

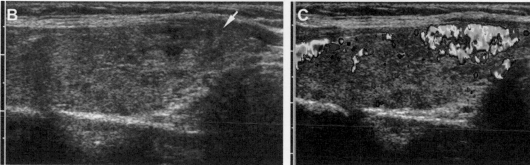

Fig. 15. Papillary carcinoma. (*A*) Transverse sonographic image of the left lobe of the thyroid in a 12-year-old boy with a palpable thyroid nodule shows an ill-defined hyperechoic mass with punctate echogenic foci suggesting microcalcifications. (*B*) Longitudinal gray-scale image of the right lobe of the thyroid in a 14-year-old girl with a palpable thyroid nodule shows an ill-defined heterogeneous hypoechoic mass (*arrow*) in the lower pole. (*C*) Color Doppler shows marked intranodular hypervascularity.

distinguishing benign and malignant thyroid lesions. The ultrasound criteria that have been found to be most reliable in identifying thyroid malignancies include irregular margins, subcapsular nodule location, and increased perinodular and intranodular vascular flow. These criteria are most useful when the nodule size is 15 mm or smaller.[71] In contradistinction to criteria commonly used for sonographic characterization of thyroid malignancies in adults, hypoechogenicity and heterogeneity show very low accuracy[71] in nodules less than or equal to 15 mm. Microcalcifications have been shown to be highly specific for thyroid malignancy in children, but have an extremely low sensitivity.[71] Although sonographic signs of cystic change in a thyroid nodule often suggest degenerating thyroid nodules, malignant thyroid lesions in children have also been shown to have cystic components, such that thyroid carcinoma should be in the differential diagnosis of a cystic thyroid nodule.[76,77]

Diffuse Thyroid Diseases

Acute suppurative thyroiditis

Acute suppurative thyroiditis is relatively rare in children due to the protective forces of the fibrous capsule, high levels of iodide within the gland, and the rich blood supply.[78] When it does occur, the typical presentation is painful enlargement of the thyroid gland in association with a euthyroid state. The infection is most commonly bacterial in origin including *Streptococcus*, *Staphylococcus*, and anaerobic bacteria. In addition, acute suppurative thyroiditis may be associated with a congenital fistula between the pyriform sinus and the ipsilateral lobe of the thyroid gland, reported to more commonly occur on the left[79,80]; this should be suspected in cases of recurrent suppurative thyroiditis.

Sonographic evaluation typically demonstrates a complex mass within the affected lobe, which may comprise one or more hypoechoic areas. Frank abscess formation may also be detected with ultrasound.

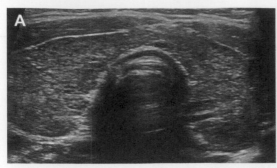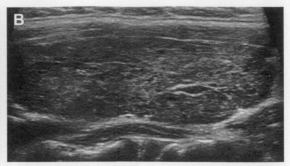

Fig. 16. Hashimoto thyroiditis. (A) Transverse and (B) longitudinal sonographic images of the thyroid gland demonstrate a diffusely enlarged gland with heterogeneous echotexture comprising multiple ill-defined hypoechoic nodules and echogenic bandlike septations.

Chronic autoimmune thyroiditis (Hashimoto thyroiditis)

Autoimmune thyroid disease is the most common cause of thyroid dysfunction in children and adolescents, and is estimated to occur in approximately 1% of school-aged children with a peak incidence during adolescence. The incidence of autoimmune thyroiditis is significantly higher in females. The pathophysiology involves lymphocytic infiltration of the thyroid gland in association with elevated circulating levels of thyroid peroxidase and thyroglobulin antibodies. Patients often present with painless enlargement of the thyroid gland, and may be euthyroid or hypothyroid. Hashimoto thyroiditis can be associated with type I diabetes and other autoimmune disorders such as celiac disease. In addition, Hashimoto thyroiditis is also associated with several chromosomal disorders such as Turner, Down, and Klinefelter syndromes.[75]

Sonographic characteristics of chronic autoimmune thyroiditis have been well established. The sonographic findings tend to evolve with time, making ultrasound a useful tool in following the disease course.[81] The classic sonographic findings include glandular enlargement with diffuse coarsening and heterogeneity of the normal echotexture, and an overall hypoechoic appearance. The presence of ill-defined small nodules thought to reflect the lymphocytic glandular infiltration creates a fine micronodular appearance. Echogenic bandlike septations may be present throughout the gland (**Fig. 16**). In the early phases of the disease process, color Doppler interrogation may reveal hypervascularity.[82] Subsequently as the disease progresses, the vascularity may be normal or decreased.

Graves disease

Graves disease, the most common cause of hyperthyroidism in children, is also autoimmune mediated, with production of thyroid-stimulating hormone receptor antibodies resulting in overproduction of thyroid hormone. On histopathology, the thyroid gland shows infiltration by lymphocytes and plasma cells and associated inflammation.

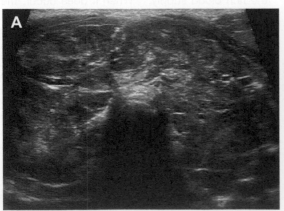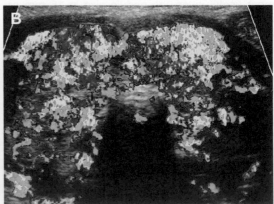

Fig. 17. Graves Disease. (A) Transverse gray-scale image of the thyroid gland demonstrates a diffusely enlarged thyroid with markedly heterogeneous echotexture. (B) Color Doppler image shows significant hyperemia.

Graves disease is rare in children, reported to occur in approximately 0.02%.[83] The incidence increases with age and peaks in adolescence, with a female predominance. Graves disease is more common in children with other autoimmune conditions and in those with a family history of autoimmune thyroid disease.[84] Clinical presentation includes variable degrees of thyroid glandular enlargement in association with the classic signs of hyperthyroidism.

Ultrasound has assumed the primary role for imaging evaluation of the thyroid gland in suspected Graves disease. Sonographic findings include symmetric thyroid enlargement to varying degrees. The thyroid contour may become lobulated. Alteration of the thyroid echotexture ranges from normal to hypoechoic, with variable heterogeneity. Color Doppler interrogation demonstrates marked hypervascularity, which has been referred to as the "thyroid inferno" (**Fig. 17**).[85]

SUMMARY

Ultrasound plays an important role in the imaging evaluation of the pediatric neck, ranging from the initial screening modality to the diagnostic tool of choice. Understanding the spectrum of disease processes affecting the pediatric neck and the associated sonographic findings is essential for the radiologist to offer a differential diagnosis, make a specific diagnosis, or suggest further imaging evaluation.

REFERENCES

1. Moore KL, Persaud TVN. The pharyngeal apparatus. The developing human. Clinically oriented embryology. 7th edition. Philadelphia: WB Saunders Co; 2003. p. 202–40.
2. Shackelford GD, McAlister WH. The aberrantly positioned thymus. A cause of mediastinal or neck masses in children. AJR Am J Roentgenol 1974; 120:291–6.
3. Tovi F, Mares AJ. The aberrant cervical thymus— embryology, pathology and clinical implications. Am J Surg 1978;136:631–7.
4. Koumanidou C, Vakaki M, Theophanopoulou M. Aberrant thymus in infants: sonographic evaluation. Pediatr Radiol 1998;28:987–9.
5. Spiegland N, Bensoussan AL, Blanchard H. Aberrant cervical thymus in children: three case reports and review of the literature. J Pediatr Surg 1990; 25:1196–9.
6. Senel S, Erkek N, Otgun I, et al. Superior herniation of the thymus into the neck—a familial pattern. J Thorac Imaging 2009;23:131–4.
7. Han BK, Babcock DS, Oestreich AE. Normal thymus in infancy: sonographic characteristics. Radiology 1989;170:471–4.
8. Han BK, Suh YL, Yoon HK. Thymic ultrasound I. Intrathymic anatomy in infants. Pediatr Radiol 2001; 31:474–9.
9. Han BK, Yoon HK, Suh YL. Thymic ultrasound II. Diagnosis of aberrant cervical thymus. Pediatr Radiol 2001;31:480–7.
10. Adam EJ, Ingotus PI. Sonography of the thymus in healthy children: frequency of visualization, size and appearance. AJR Am J Roentgenol 1993;161: 153–5.
11. Castellote A, Vaxquez E, Vera J, et al. Cervicothoracic lesions in infants and children. Radiographics 1999;19:583–600.
12. Zarbo RJ. Thymopharyngeal duct cyst: a form of cervical thymus. Ann Otol Rhinol Laryngol 1983;92: 284–8.
13. Kaufman MR, Smith S, Rothschild MA, et al. Thymopharyngeal duct cyst an unusual variant of cervical thymic anomalies. Arch Otolarynol Head Neck Surg 2001;127:1357–60.
14. Siegel MJ. Pediatric sonography. 3rd edition. Philadelphia: Lippincott Williams and Wilkins; 2002.
15. Kutuya N, Kurosaki Y. Sonographic assessment of thyroglossal duct cysts in children. J Ultrasound Med 2008;27:1211–9.
16. Wadsworth DT, Siegel MJ. Thyroglossal duct cysts: variability of sonographic findings. AJR Am J Roentgenol 1994;163:1475–7.
17. Ahuja AT, King AD, Metreweli C. Sonographic evaluation of thyroglossal duct cysts in children. Clin Radiol 2000;55:770–4.
18. Saiki JH. Severe myxedema following inadvertent removal of an ectopic thyroid resembling a thyroglossal duct cyst. Lancet 1967;87:7–9.
19. Noyek AM, Friedberg J. Thyroglossal duct and ectopic thyroid disorders. Otolaryngol Clin North Am 1981;14:187–201.
20. Lin-Dunham JE, Feinstein KA, Yousefzadeh DK, et al. Sonographic demonstration of a normal thyroid gland excludes ectopic thyroid in patients with thyroglossal duct cyst. AJR Am J Roentgenol 1995; 164:1489 91.
21. Yasumoto M, Shibuya H, Gomi N, et al. Ultrasonographic appearance of dermoid and epidermoid cysts in the head and neck. J Clin Ultrasound 1991;19:455–61.
22. Vazquez E, Enriquez G, Castellote A, et al. US, CT and MR imaging of neck lesions in children. Radiographics 1995;15:105–22.
23. Elmasalme F, Giacomantonio M, Clark KD, et al. Congenital cervical teratoma in neonates case report and review. Eur J Pediatr Surg 2000;10: 252–7.

24. Koeller KK, Alamo L, Adair CF, et al. Congenital cystic masses of the neck: radiologic pathologic correlation. Radiographics 1999;19:121–46.

25. Waldenhausen JHT. Branchial cleft and arch anomalies in children. Semin Pediatr Surg 2006; 15:64–9.

26. Koch B. Cystic malformations of the neck in children. Pediatr Radiol 2005;35:463–77.

27. Reynolds JH, Wolinski AP. Sonographic appearance of branchial cysts. Clin Radiol 1993;48: 109–10.

28. Gonzales J, Ljung B, Guerry T, et al. Congenital torticollis: evaluation by fine needle aspiration biopsy. Laryngoscope 1989;99:651–4.

29. Chan YL, Cheng JC, Metreweli C. Ultrasound of congenital muscular torticollis. Pediatr Radiol 1992; 22:356–60.

30. Crawford SC, Hamberger HR, Johnson L, et al. Fibromatosis colli of infancy: CT and sonographic findings. AJR Am J Roentgenol 1988;151:1183–4.

31. Ablin DS, Jain K, Howell L, et al. Ultrasound and MR imaging of fibromatosis colli (sternocleidomastoid tumor of infancy). Pediatr Radiol 1998;28: 230–3.

32. Lin JN, Chou ML. Ultrasonographic study of the sternocleidomastoid muscle in the management of congenital muscular torticollis. J Pediatr Surg 1997;32:1648–51.

33. Bedi DG, John SD, Swischuk LE. Fibromatosis colli of infancy: variability of sonographic appearance. J Clin Ultrasound 1998;26:345–8.

34. Gosche JR, Vick L. Acute, subacute, and chronic cervical lymphadenitis in children. Semin Pediatr Surg 2006;15:99–106.

35. Leung AKC, Davies HD. Cervical lymphadenitis: etiology, diagnosis, and management. Curr Infect Dis Rep 2009;11:183–9.

36. Papakonstantinou O, Bakantaki A, Paspalaki P, et al. High-resolution and color Doppler ultrasonography of cervical lymphadenopathy in children. Acta Radiol 2001;42:470–6.

37. Niedzielska G, Kotowski M, Niedzielski A, et al. Cervical lymphadenopathy in children—incidence and diagnostic management. Int J Pediatr Otorhinolaryngol 2007;71:51–6.

38. Douglas SA, Jennings S, Owen VMF, et al. Is ultrasound useful for evaluating pediatric inflammatory neck masses? Clin Otolaryngol 2005;30: 526–9.

39. Dulin MF, Kennard TP, Leach L. Management of cervical lymphadenitis in children. Am Fam Physician 2008;78:1097–8.

40. Finn MD, Glowacki J, Mulliken JB. Congenital vascular lesions: clinical application of a new classification. J Pediatr Surg 1983;18:894–9.

41. Mulliken JB, Glowacki J. Hemangiomas and vascular malformations in infants and children:

42. Paltiel HJ, Burrows PE, Kozakewich HPW, et al. Soft tissue vascular anomalies: utility of US for diagnosis. Radiology 2000;214:747–54.

43. Dubois J, Patriquin HB, Garel L, et al. Soft tissue hemangiomas in infants and children: diagnosis using Doppler sonography. AJR Am J Roentgenol 1998;171:247–52.

44. Dubois J, Garel L, David M, et al. Vascular soft tissue tumors in infancy: distinguishing features on Doppler sonography. AJR Am J Roentgenol 2002; 178:1541–5.

45. Ahuja AT, Richards P, Wong KT, et al. Accuracy of high-resolution sonography compared with magnetic resonance imaging in the diagnosis of head and neck venous vascular malformations. Clin Radiol 2003;58:869–75.

46. Yang WT, Ahuja A, Metreweli C. Sonographic features of head and neck hemangiomas and vascular malformations: review of 23 patients. J Ultrasound Med 1997;16:39–44.

47. Flis C, Connor S. Imaging of head and neck venous malformations. Eur Radiol 2005;15:2185–93.

48. Ahuja AT, Ying M, Ho SY, et al. Ultrasound of malignant cervical lymph nodes. Cancer Imaging 2008;8:48–56.

49. Ying M, Ahuja A, Brook F. Accuracy of sonographic vascular features in differentiating different causes of cervical lymphadenopathy. Ultrasound Med Biol 2004;30:441–7.

50. Sebire NJ, Roebuck DJ. Pathological diagnosis of paediatric tumours from image-guided needle core biopsies: a systematic review. Pediatr Radiol 2006; 36:426–31.

51. Kraus R, Han BK, Babcock DS, et al. Sonography of neck masses in children. AJR Am J Roentgenol 1986;146:609–13.

52. Van Rijn RR, Wilde JC, Bras J, et al. Imaging findings in noncraniofacial childhood rhabdomyosarcoma. Pediatr Radiol 2008;38:617–34.

53. Abramson SJ, Berdon WE, Ruzal-Shapiro C, et al. Cervical neuroblastoma in eleven infants—a tumor with favorable prognosis. Pediatr Radiol 1993;23: 253–7.

54. Kojima K, Thomas R, Silberberg P. Pediatric radiology normal measurements website. Available at: http://www.ohsu.edu/radiology/teach/kojima/thyroid. htm. Accessed August 14, 2009.

55. Ueda D. Normal volume of the thyroid gland in children. J Clin Ultrasound 1990;18:455–62.

56. Vade A, Gottschalk ME, Etter EM. Sonographic measurements of the neonatal thyroid gland. J Ultrasound Med 1997;16:395–9.

57. Perry RJ, Hollman AS, Wood AM, et al. Ultrasound of the thyroid gland in the newborn: normative data. Arch Dis Child Fetal Neonatal Ed 2002;87: F209–11.

a classification based on endothelial characteristics. Plast Reconstr Surg 1982;69:412–22.

58. Buyukgebiz A. Newborn screening for congenital hypothyroidism. J Pediatr Endocrinol Metab 2006; 19:1291–8.

59. Devos H, Rodd C, Gagne N, et al. A search for the possible mechanisms of thyroid dysgenesis: sex ratios and associated malformations. J Clin Endocrinol Metab 1999;84:2502–6.

60. Ogawa E, Kanako KI, Ikuma F. Ultrasound appearance of thyroid tissue in hypothyroid infants. J Pediatr 2008;153:101–4.

61. Takashima S, Nomura N, Tanaka H, et al. Congenital hypothyroidism: assessment with ultrasound. AJNR Am J Neuroradiol 1995;16:1117–23.

62. Ohnishi H, Sato H, Noda H, et al. Color Doppler ultrasonography: diagnosis of ectopic thyroid gland in patients with congenital hypothyroidism caused by thyroid dysgenesis. J Clin Endocrinol Metab 2003;88:5145–9.

63. Rallison ML, Brown MD, Keating FR, et al. Thyroid nodularity in children. JAMA 1975;233:1069–72.

64. Yip FWK, Reeve TS, Poole AG, et al. Thyroid nodules in childhood and adolescence. Aust N Z J Surg 1994;64:676–8.

65. Hung W. Solitary thyroid nodules in 93 children and adolescents. Horm Res 1999;52:15–8.

66. Babcock DS. Thyroid disease in the pediatric patient: emphasizing imaging with sonography. Pediatr Radiol 2006;36:299–308.

67. Solbiati L, Charboneau JW, Osti V, et al. The thyroid gland. In: Rumack CM, Wilson SR, Charboneau JW, et al, editors. Diagnostic ultrasound. 3rd edition. St. Louis (MO): Elsevier Mosby; 2004. p. 735–70.

68. Zohar Y, Strauss M, Laurian N. Adolescent versus adult thyroid carcinoma. Laryngoscope 1986;96: 555–9.

69. Raab SS, Silverman JF, Elsheikh TM, et al. Pediatric thyroid nodules: disease demographics and clinical management as determined by fine needle aspiration. Pediatrics 1995;95:46–9.

70. Bucsky P, Parlowsky T. Epidemiology and therapy of thyroid cancer in childhood and adolescence. Exp Clin Endocrinol Diabetes 1997;105(Suppl 4): 70–3.

71. Lyshchik A, Drozd V, Demidchik Y. Diagnosis of thyroid cancer in children: value of gray-scale and power Doppler US. Radiology 2005;235:604–13.

72. Goepfert H, Dichtel WJ, Samaan NA. Thyroid cancer in children and teenagers. Arch Otolaryngol 1984; 110:72–5.

73. Grigsby PW, Gal-or A, Michalski JM, et al. Childhood and adolescent thyroid carcinoma. Cancer 2002;95: 724–9.

74. Massimino M, Gasparini M, Ballerini E, et al. Primary thyroid carcinoma in children: a retrospective study of 20 patients. Med Pediatr Oncol 1995;24:13–7.

75. Behrmann RE, Kliegman RM, Jenson HB. Neson textbook of pediatrics. Philadelphia: Saunders; 2004.

76. Yoskovitch A, Laberge JM, Rodd C, et al. Cystic thyroid lesions in children. J Pediatr Surg 1998;33: 866–70.

77. Desjardin JG, Khan AH, Montupet P, et al. Management of thyroid nodules in children. A 20-year experience. J Pediatr Surg 1987;22:736–9.

78. Hsin C, Lee YJ, Chiu NC, et al. Acute suppurative thyroiditis in children. Pediatr Infect Dis J 2002;21: 384–7.

79. Lucaya J, Berdon WE, Enriquez G, et al. Congenital pyriform sinus fistula: a cause of acute left-sided suppurative thyroiditis and neck abscess in children. Pediatr Radiol 1990;21:27–9.

80. Ahuja AT, Griffiths JF, Roebuck WK, et al. The role of ultrasound and oesophagography in the management of acute suppurative thyroiditis in children associated with congenital pyriform fossa sinus. Clin Radiol 1998;53:209–11.

81. Vlachopapadopoulou E, Thomas D, Karachaliou F, et al. Evolution of sonographic appearance of the thyroid gland in children with Hashimoto's thyroiditis. J Pediatr Endocrinol Metab 2009;22:339–44.

82. Toma P, Rossi UG, Magnaguagno F, et al. Imaging of the normal and affected thyroid in children with emphasis on sonography. Pediatr Endocrinol Rev 2003;1:237–43.

83. Kaguelidou F, Carel JC, Leger J. Graves' disease in childhood: advances in management with antithyroid drug therapy. Horm Res 2009; 71:310–7.

84. Cooper DS. Hyperthyroidism. Lancet 2003;362: 459–68.

85. Ralls PW, Mayekawa DS, lee KP, et al. Color-flow Doppler sonography in Graves disease: "thyroid inferno". AJR Am J Roentgenol 1988;150:781–4.

Index

Note: Page numbers of article titles are in **boldface** type.

Ultrasound Clin 4 (2009) 571–576
doi:10.1016/S1556-858X(09)00103-0

Printed and bound by CPI Group (UK) Ltd, Croydon, CR0 4YY

03/10/2024

01040353-0004